ADAM GAVINE & ROD BONELLO

BACK PAIN

HOW TO BUILD CORE STABILITY FOR LONG-LASTING RELIEF

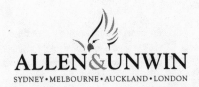

ALLEN&UNWIN

SYDNEY · MELBOURNE · AUCKLAND · LONDON

First published in 2014

Allen & Unwin
83 Alexander Street
Crows Nest NSW 2065
Australia
Phone: (61 2) 8425 0100
Email: info@allenandunwin.com
Web: www.allenandunwin.com

Cataloguing-in-Publication details are available
from the National Library of Australia
www.trove.nla.gov.au

ISBN 978 1 74331 712 9

Illustrations by Ian Faulkner, www.ianfaulknerillustrator.com
Set in 12/15 pt Adobe Garamond by Midland Typesetters, Australia
Printed and bound in Australia by Griffin Press

10 9 8 7 6 5 4 3 2 1

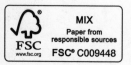

Contents

Contents

Contents

Preface

Today the importance of the spine in health and disease is widely appreciated. Looking after your spine is an important strategy in avoiding back pain and in gaining health and wellbeing. Chiropractors and other health professionals have developed skills and expertise in helping people with spinal problems. In an ideal world health professionals should be coaches, helping their patients get the best performance out of their bodies, rather than therapists patching people together again.

Healthcare costs are escalating and the best defense against this situation is when people take responsibility for their own wellbeing. Following sound advice and having a periodic check up is far better than waiting until things to start to fall apart. Self-help strategies will not always replace the care offered by a clinical expert but they should minimise the need for care and can speed up recovery.

Martin Harvey BSc (Anat), MChiro
President, Australian Spinal Research Foundation

Introduction

The spine is one of the most complex and misunderstood structures in the body. It is comprised of muscles, bones, ligaments, joints, nerves and numerous other tissue types. As a result of its complexity identifying the exact cause of back pain can be exceptionally difficult.

Most people with back pain have a simple sprain/strain type of injury that is often related to poor movement of the spine (biomechanics). However, rarely back pain can be caused by serious damage or disease, which is why it is important to have it thoroughly investigated by a health professional with detailed knowledge of the spine.

Back pain can be triggered by everyday activities at work or at home, or during other activities. Often back pain can be due to an underlying condition that has been gradually developing over time, sometimes years or even decades. Sometimes the final event that triggers the onset of pain is trivial (for example, bending to pick up a newspaper, coughing or sneezing). Some common causes of back pain include:

- poor posture
- incorrect bending or moving
- incorrect lifting, carrying, pushing or pulling
- slouching in chairs
- standing or bending down for long periods
- overstretching or twisting too far
- sustained driving without taking a break
- overuse activities, usually due to sport or repetitive movements
- lifestyle and mental stress.

This book provides information on the nature of back pain, the physical structures involved, disorders of the back, factors that aggravate back pain, methods of assessing and diagnosing back pain, as well as current available treatments.

Treat the cause, not the symptom

If the cause of an injury or dysfunction is not addressed, the results of treatment will be temporary at best. Many practitioners fail to give patients great results because they treat the symptoms and not the cause. Any practitioner can easily treat your symptoms; we simply ask you to point to where it hurts and treat that area. A good practitioner will endeavour to figure out why it hurts at that particular location, and fix the *cause* of the symptoms. This approach provides superior results and a lasting effect!

How big is this issue?

Back pain is a major economic problem and has significant costs for individuals and our healthcare system, as well as absenteeism from work. Close to 80 per cent of us will have substantial back pain at some time in our lives. This is known as the lifetime prevalence of back pain. It is estimated that 15 per cent to 20 per cent of the population experiences low back pain annually (the point prevalence). At any given time, 2 per cent of the population is disabled because of back problems. Historically, low back pain has been the second-leading cause of outpatient visits to doctors and therapists, and is the most common reason for visits to chiropractors, physiotherapists, osteopaths and massage therapists.

The Global Burden of Disease Study ranked low back pain as the sixth-worst problem globally in terms of causing disability. Amazingly, in Australia, low back pain was ranked as *the worst problem*, and neck pain was 10th in terms of disability.

It has been estimated that the cost of low back pain in Australia is over $1 billion for direct costs (including treatment and compensation costs) but over $8 billion in indirect costs (such as loss of production, replacement staff costs, administration costs and reduced productivity). In any six-month period approximately 10 per cent of Australian adults suffer some significant disability from low back pain. A 2013 WHO report identified low back pain as the number one cause of disability worldwide.

The Australian Institute of Health and Welfare reported:

- The Australian Bureau of Statistics 2007–08 National Health Survey estimates that about 1.8 million Australians (9.2 per cent of the population) have current back problems.
- Back problems are a common reason for pain among younger and middle-aged adults, but they can start early in life (between ages 8 and 10).
- For long-term back problem sufferers, 14 per cent experience constant or persistent pain and 86 per cent experience pain one day per week.
- According to the National Hospital Morbidity Database, in 2010–11 there were 93,564 hospitalisations with a principal diagnosis of back problems. The common reasons for hospitalisations were:
  - low back pain (27.7 per cent of hospitalisations for back problems)
  - narrowing of the spinal canal, or **spinal stenosis** (14.1 per cent)
  - pain including tingling, numbness and weakness in the legs that starts from the lower back, or sciatica (13.8 per cent).

Why practitioners fail to fix chronic low back pain

A major reason practitioners fail to resolve chronic low back pain is because they fail to nail down an accurate diagnosis. No specific medical diagnosis is made in approximately 90 per cent of low back pain patients. Often this is because most causes of low back pain lack objective clinical signs and overt pathological changes. Over 70 per cent of all chronic low back pain comes from either a facet joint, sacroiliac joint or disc. So why are practitioners still not coming up with a diagnosis for patients with chronic low back pain? The purpose of a diagnosis is to identify a condition and its specific location. If a diagnosis fails to do so, it is worthless. If you are given a specific diagnosis, you have a much better chance of seeing results from a tailored treatment.

When practitioners are unsuccessful in improving low back pain it usually means one of two things. Either their diagnosis is wrong and, therefore, their treatment is inappropriate, or the diagnosis is correct but the practitioner is not skilled enough to fix the problem. With an experienced practitioner, the likelihood of their skill being inadequate decreases dramatically. Therefore, the most common cause of treatment failure is an incorrect diagnosis. Don't be afraid to ask your practitioner to tell you what your diagnosis is. Even better, ask them to write it down for you.

Pain

Pain is a confusing concept, and one that we still don't fully understand. Pain is defined by the International Association for the Study of Pain as an unpleasant sensory and emotional experience associated with actual or potential tissue damage. Pain is how your body lets you know something is not right. Issues often arise when we choose to ignore pain or take drugs to numb the effects of pain.

Medicine, allied health care and complementary medicine

Luckily, you have a wide choice in the type of health practitioner you can consult for your health needs. It's been reported that 42 per cent of the population in the United States now use non-medical approaches such as complementary or alternative medicine, especially for back problems. Chiropractic treatment was reported to be the most popular of the 16 alternative therapies examined. Another study reported that 54 per cent of the population in the United States use complementary or alternative medicine, of which chiropractic treatment accounted for 20 per cent, massage for 14 per cent and relaxation techniques accounted for 12 per cent of treatments. Standard medical treatment providers were rated 'very helpful' for back and neck pain by 27 per cent of patients. In comparison, up to 65 per cent of complementary and alternative treatment seekers rated those therapies as 'very helpful'.

How to use this book

If you have a back problem or wish to avoid back problems, this book is for you. It's written to explain back problems and what to do about them. If you currently have back pain, this book will help you get the most out of the treatments you are having and advise you on what you can do at home to facilitate your recovery. We start with spine anatomy because most back problems are mechanical (not disease-related). If you understand how the back works, you can optimise its recovery. Knowing the terminology will also help you unravel what may otherwise be very difficult to understand.

The second chapter covers details of conditions which affect the back. If you have been diagnosed, this is where you can find your problem explained. Chapter 3 reviews the diagnostic process. Often people with back pain endure prolonged suffering because they have never been diagnosed properly. Chapter 4 outlines the most commonly used treatments for back pain, and includes both invasive and non-invasive therapies. Chapter 5 provides a guide on how to choose a good practitioner. Most back pain sufferers need to be managed by more than one kind of practitioner. This chapter helps you choose the best ones for you. Chapter 6 looks at back pain in the workplace. It covers both causes and prevention of back pain at work, and also how to manage work when you have back pain. Chapter 7 covers many Dos and Don'ts for looking after your back—whether you have a back problem or not. If you do have one, we have included a colour section that contains strategies to help you move more comfortably. In the same section we cover exercises and self-mobilisations that can rehabilitate mechanical-related back pain and help prevent back pain in most people.

We provide a glossary to help you understand the anatomical and other technical terms used in this book. Glossary words are written in **bold** in the text. We list references to the sources of knowledge that are the basis of the ideas of this book. As we believe in evidence-based approaches as the best strategies in health care we feel it's crucial to show you the evidence rather than expect you to take this advice because it is written here. If you wish, you can go to the source of the information to explore the issues in more detail.

Guide to the rehabilitation exercises

The following instructions will help you get the most value from the colour exercise section in this book.

Research shows that exercise therapy and mobilisations are a safe and effective component in the management of most back problems. Exercises for core stability are believed to be protective, preventative and rehabilitative for back problems. This section has been designed to be a self-help guide to introduce you to active mobilisations and help you to develop your core stability in a safe and progressive manner. Most texts on the subject of core-stability training offer many variations of exercises, but very few of them actually discuss where or how to begin. Fewer still describe in detail a logical progression for each exercise and almost none of them describe which exercises are safe to perform and which are contraindicated for certain people. The inappropriate use of exercise therapy can be dangerous, as it can perpetuate your back condition or, even worse, exacerbate your condition. By addressing these issues in this book we have attempted to deal with some of the shortcomings of other texts. We want you to have a clear and concise understanding of how to use these exercises. When the appropriate exercises are selected for the right circumstances, and done correctly, the results can be astounding.

The four sides of the torso form the cylindrical shape of the core stability muscle group. They are: the **anterior**, **posterior**, and two **lateral** aspects of the torso. Our core muscles are only as strong as the weakest link. So doing exercises that work the anterior and lateral sections but fail to train the posterior muscles will leave you weak in the posterior muscles and compromise the integrity of the entire core. Therefore, in order to avoid any chinks in your armour, you need to train each section appropriately to attain balanced function. This does not imply that you should work each section equally—this may be the case for some, but for others a particular section make be inherently weak and require more training to bring it on par with the other sections. It shouldn't be difficult to figure out if you are weaker in one section. A simple way to diagnose your weak section is to assess which exercise you struggle with the most or feel weakest while performing. A more objective method is to test your core endurance for each section (for a complete description of each test, refer to the exercise pages).

We recommend performing all three endurance tests and logging your results before you start your core-stability training in earnest. The results provide a useful benchmark for you to objectively assess your progression. Say you are able to hold the 'anterior core endurance test' for 20 seconds in Week 1. If when you retest yourself in Week 5 you improve your hold time to 30 seconds, that's a significant improvement. Generally people tend to improve their hold times more dramatically in the first few weeks of the training protocol, so don't be disappointed if after you've been doing the exercises for a few months your times don't increase by as much; this is normal. If you fail to increase you hold times after several weeks of performing the exercises regularly, we recommend you consult your practitioner or someone knowledgeable and experienced in these exercises to assess whether you are performing the exercises properly. Another reason could be that you are simply not performing the exercises regularly enough. Also, consider internal factors—if you are ill, stressed out or run down, your body will fail to respond in an appropriate manner and your results may reflect this. You may need to get more sleep, take some time off work or minimise exercise until you are better. Lastly, external factors can negatively influence your results as well. For example, you are performing a new manual task at work that irritates your back, or you are using a new chair that is not appropriate for your back. These issues can negatively influence your training results, because they limit your ability to perform the exercises effectively. Therefore, we recommend regularly reassessing such factors and taking the appropriate actions to rectify any issues to achieve the best possible results from your core stability training.

Exercise therapy involves exercises being repeated in certain patterns. The number of times an exercise is repeated is called the repetitions or 'reps'. So, an exercise which is performed six times in a row is said to have six reps. For exercise therapy to be effective, usually the reps have to be performed a few times. These are called sets. So if you perform your exercise of six reps twice over, that would be two sets of six reps. This is not the same as performing that exercise 12 times in a row as a short spell or breather is taken between sets. Alternately, a different exercise may be performed in between sets. This allows for the exercise routine to be performed without fatiguing the target muscles.

Each exercise has been written with a basic default starting point in regard to the number sets and reps to be performed. To facilitate progression we recommend you increase the number of reps by 2–5 reps when you feel as though you can complete the default sets and reps with relative ease. Continue to increase the number of reps until you are performing two sets of 15 reps (30 total reps). To progress further, we advise you to now increase the number of sets but drop the number of repetitions to keep the total number of repetitions relatively close. In this example the progression would be to do three sets of 8–10 reps (24–30 total reps). It should be noted that performing more sets is generally harder than performing more repetitions. You can work your way up to doing a maximum of 15 repetitions, at which point you would again increase the number of sets to four and again reduce to 8–10 reps. This procedure can be followed until you reach a maximum of four sets of 15 reps, at which point you can graduate to the next difficulty level for that exercise.

For those exercises which require you to hold a position for a specified duration, we suggest increasing the hold time progressively by 5 second increments. After you have reached a 20 second hold you can increase the number of repetitions. The following table is an example of how this can be done.

Bird dog beginner exercise

Week 1 2 sets of 15 reps
Week 2 3 sets of 10 reps
Week 3 3 sets of 15 reps
Week 4 4 sets of 10 reps
Week 5 4 sets of 15 reps
Week 6 Graduate to Bird dog intermediate exercise starting with 3 sets of 10 reps

In order to facilitate a safe and easy progression for each exercise we use the star rating system. The one-star rating is the easiest form of the exercise, and a five-star rating is the hardest or most difficult form of the exercise. It is not necessary to begin with the easiest star level: for some individuals, the

Front plank intermediate exercise

Week 1   2 sets of 2 reps holding for 15 seconds each time
Week 2   2 sets of 2 reps holding for 20 seconds each time
Week 3   2 sets of 3 reps holding for 15 seconds each time
Week 4   2 sets of 3 reps holding for 20 seconds each time
Week 5   2 sets of 4 reps holding for 15 seconds each time
Week 6   2 sets of 4 reps holding for 20 seconds each time
Week 7   Graduate to Front plank advanced exercise starting with 2 sets of
          2 reps holding for 15 seconds each time.

exercise will be far too easy and no physical improvements will be achieved by doing them. An easy way to assess whether you belong at a specific star level is to see if you can easily perform four sets of 15 reps of the exercise. If you can, then it is safe to say you should begin at a higher star level.

Similarly, once you have progressed in an exercise and reached the limit of four sets of 15 reps, it is time to move up an exercise star ranking (for example, move from a two-star exercise to a three-star exercise).

Finally, we have colour-coded and labelled each exercise according to what section of the core it focuses on. Every exercise in this chapter will fall under one of the following headings: anterior, posterior or lateral core stability. In order to have a balanced core, we recommend selecting at least one exercise from each of these headings (one anterior exercise, one posterior exercise and one lateral exercise). You may decide to do more than one exercise for one section, but be careful not to overwork one section and under-develop another. As you progress with the exercises, try switching some of the exercises around to keep things interesting (many of the exercises have alternative versions of the same exercise for the same star level).

When examining the effects of mobilisations, all of them affect the nerves to some degree; however, certain mobilisations have been developed that specifically target the nerves. These mobilisations are forms of 'nerve flossing'. Nerve flossing involves tensioning one end of a nerve and simultaneously slackening the opposite end while actively moving through a range of motion. The aim is to free up entrapped nerves by flossing them 'to and fro' past an adhesion (sticking point).

We wish to give you guidelines to follow, but we don't want to be taskmasters. We recommend performing these exercises daily if possible; however, doing them three times per week is the minimum requirement to get effective results. If you can't be bothered doing all the exercises on your training day, that's OK. Just try doing one exercise instead; it's better than doing none at all. You have to start somewhere, so if you are experiencing severe back pain or are unmotivated, that would be a good starting point. After a few weeks you will likely find it easier to do that one exercise and you may decide to go for two exercises, and then the next week, three exercises—it snowballs from there. Eventually you will work up to doing all three areas of the core, at which point you will really begin to notice the improvements.

Remember these exercises don't have to be arduous and boring. Try making the exercises fun by playing your favourite music while you do them or get your partner or kids to do them with you. You can even set up a competition with your family or friends to see who has the longest time on the endurance tests after a set number of weeks of training.

We hope these exercises will help you achieve your goals on your road to recovery from back pain. Our system should allow you to easily figure out a good starting point, and allow you to progress in a clear and steady manner. However, if you still feel unsure about where to begin, or are concerned about your form while performing the exercises, we recommend consulting with a knowledgeable therapist or trainer who can help you answer these questions. If you don't know a good therapist or trainer, refer to Chapter 5.

If you'd like further information, we are in the process of developing a smartphone app that includes an accompanying video explanation of each exercise outlined in this book.

Safety notice

If any exercise causes or aggravates your pain, you must stop that exercise immediately. Exercise therapy can be strenuous but it should not exacerbate your pain or have you push through a pain barrier. Doing that will probably make your back problem worsen or just cause unnecessary pain. An exception is the McKenzie exercises in the colour section, which do involve discomfort or mild pain during their performance. As always, if in doubt, consult a therapist.

Although we hope you will enjoy reading this book, more importantly, we trust that it will give you strategies to understand and control your back issues so that they no longer limit what you do.

1 Anatomy

A thorough knowledge of anatomy is fundamental for healthcare workers, and we think that some knowledge in this area would be useful to you too. If you're really not interested in this section, you can skip it—you can always come back to it later.

Spinal column

The human spinal column is made up of 33 individual bones, called vertebrae, and 23 intervertebral discs. The column is divided into five regions: cervical, thoracic, lumbar, sacral and coccygeal. Adults have seven cervical, twelve thoracic, five lumbar, five sacral and four coccygeal vertebrae. We are born with five sacral and four coccygeal vertebrae, these eventually fuse to form the sacrum and the coccyx in adulthood. The fusion process begins around 16 years of age and is usually completed by the age of 26. The spinal column provides a base of support for the head and internal organs, protects the spinal cord, and provides an attachment point for ligaments, bones, muscles, the rib cage and the pelvis. It serves as a linkage between the upper and lower extremities.

No two vertebrae are exactly alike. The size of the vertebrae and their corresponding intervertebral discs increase progressively from the cervical to the lumbar spine, due to the fact that the (lower) lumbar spine is required to bear greater loads. There are five transitional areas in the spine. Starting from the head they are the atlanto-occipital joint, the cervico-thoracic junction, the thoraco-lumbar junction, the lumbo-sacral junction and sacro-coccygeal joint. Transitional areas of the spine are

Spinal Column: Lateral (Side) and Posterior (Back) Views

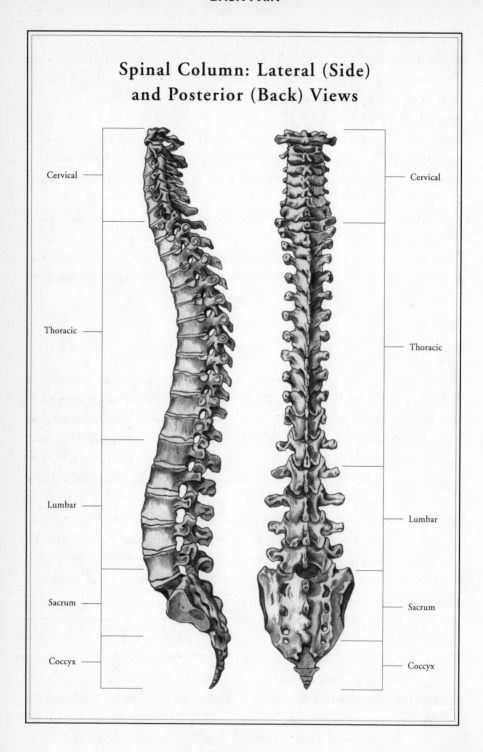

Cervical

Thoracic

Lumbar

Sacrum

Coccyx

Cervical

Thoracic

Lumbar

Sacrum

Coccyx

areas where individual vertebrae and vertebral curves change from one shape to another. This generally occurs over the course of a few vertebrae. The cervico-thoracic junction, for example, is where the spine changes from a cervical to a thoracic vertebrae (C7–T1). Transitional areas, as a general rule, have less range of motion than other areas of the spine. That is why they are often areas of interest when the spine is being treated by a practitioner. It is possible to have an extra vertebra or one too few due to a congenital anomaly. This most commonly occurs in transitional areas of the spine.

When viewed from behind (**posterior**), the spine ideally should appear in a straight vertical line. Any **lateral** curvature of the spine when viewed from behind is abnormal and is commonly referred to as a **scoliosis**; however, the lateral curvature must be at least 10 degrees curve radius to be deemed a true scoliosis.

Spinal curves

We are born with only one spinal curve, termed 'the primary curve'. It is a posterior or backward facing convex curve referred to as a **kyphosis**. During our first year of life, a secondary curve, which is forward or **anteriorly** convex (like the back of a spoon), termed a **lordosis**, begins to appear due to muscle development. The first lordosis begins to develop in utero, (as early as the seventh week) but does not become functional until the infant is able to hold the head upright. A second lordosis starts to form in the lumbar spine when the infant begins to push up when lying on its stomach. These two secondary curves continue to develop until growth stops at between 12 and 17 years of age.

When viewed from the side, the adult spine has a total of four anterior–posterior curves: two kyphoses (thoracic and sacral) and two lordoses (cervical and lumbar). While the degree of curvature varies from each section of the spine, there is a range for each section that is considered normal. Excessive or diminished spinal curves lead to adverse biomechanical and postural changes. Excessive curvature in the cervical or lumbar spine is referred to as hyperlordotic, while diminished curvature is referred to as hypolordotic. The same holds true with kyphotic curves: excessive = hyperkyphotic; diminished = hypokyphotic. Certain conditions cause

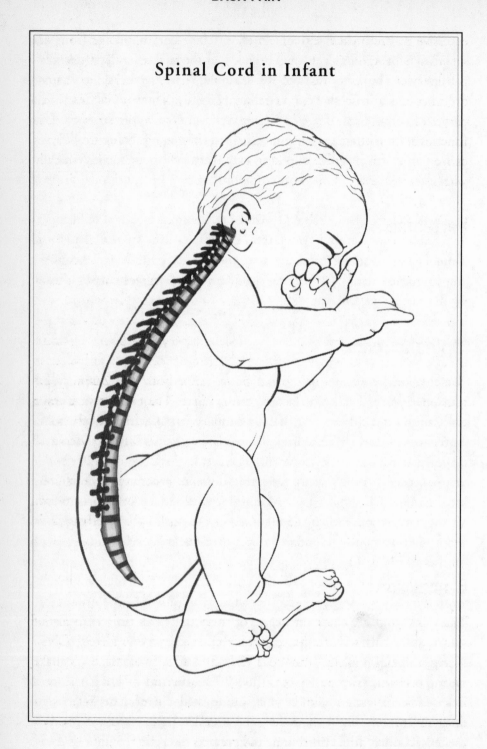

Spinal Cord in Infant

excessive or diminished curves. A few of these common conditions are scoliosis, Scheuermann's disease, ankylosing spondylitis and diffuse idiopathic skeletal hyperostosis (DISH). All spinal curves are either 'structural' or 'functional'. Structural curves are unable to straighten while functional curves can straighten. The good news is that if your hyper/hypo curve is functional (not structural), it can be helped more easily. Structural curves can only be straightened with surgery, but can be treated mechanically with some success.

Vertebrae

Vertebrae, or vertebral segments, are the bony components of the spine. The human spine has 33 vertebrae. Each lumbar vertebral segment is composed of a vertebral body anteriorly, and the posterior elements at the rear. The vertebral body is the thick, box-like structure that sits between the intervertebral discs. It is bordered by the anterior longitudinal ligament in front and the posterior longitudinal ligament behind. The posterior elements include the pedicles that support lateral bony protrusions called transverse processes that connect to the laminae. The two laminae come together to form the bits that you can see or feel in the centre of the back. At the top and bottom these laminae are the superior articular processes of the lower vertebra that connects with the **inferior** articular processes of the vertebra directly above it. The internal girder-like structures made of bone are the trabeculae, which are found in a vertical or horizontal orientation. This crisscross patterning of trabeculae is what gives the vertebrae their tremendous strength and compressibility (see picture).

Spinal cord

The spinal cord is a thick cord of nerve tissue that gives rise to 31 pairs of spinal nerves and, with the brain, forms the central nervous system (CNS). Nerves that begin at the spinal cord and travel throughout the body make up the peripheral nervous system (PNS). The diameter of the spinal cord is approximately the thickness of a human adult finger. The spinal cord descends from the brain along the spine within a narrow passageway called the central canal, which surrounds and protects the delicate spinal cord.

Top and Side Views of Vertebrae

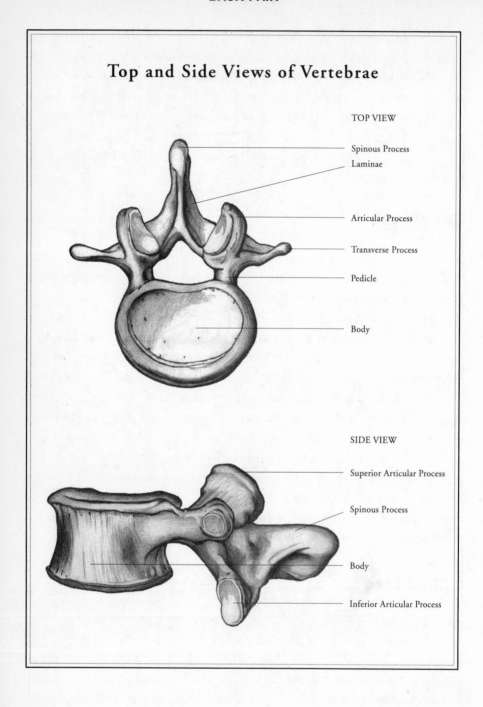

TOP VIEW

Spinous Process
Laminae

Articular Process

Transverse Process

Pedicle

Body

SIDE VIEW

Superior Articular Process

Spinous Process

Body

Inferior Articular Process

Relation of Spinal Nerve Roots to Vertebrae

Base of Skull

Cervical enlargement

C7

T7

Lumbar enlargement

L1

Conus medullaris

Cauda equina

Termination of dural sac

The spinal cord is bathed in a clear fluid called cerebral spinal fluid (CSF), which cushions the cord during movement. The function of the spinal cord is to transmit electrical information to and from the limbs, trunk and organs of the body, as well as to and from the brain. The nerves that carry information from the body to the brain are called sensory nerves, and they relay information to the brain regarding skin temperature, touch, pain and joint position. The nerves that carry information from the brain to the body are called motor nerves; they send signals that control muscles. The spinal nerves exit the spine through small bony windows called intervertebral foramina.

As a unit, the spinal cord actually ends between the L1 and L2 lumbar vertebrae. The spinal cord then separates into a fine bundle of remaining spinal nerves called the cauda equina, which literally means 'horses hair' because of its resemblance. The far end of the cauda equina is tethered to the tip of the coccyx.

Meninges

The spinal cord is covered by a system of membranes called meninges. The primary function of the meninges is to protect the central nervous system (spinal cord and brain). The meninges are fused to the spinal nerves and end where the spinal nerves begin just outside the intervertebral foramina (see diagram). There are three meningeal layers. The outermost layer is made up of dense fibrous tissue providing a protective barrier. The middle layer cushions the spinal cord and attaches to the inner layer, which is a thin transparent membrane composed of fibrous tissue. The deepest layer firmly adheres to the surface of the spinal cord.

Infection of the meninges, called meningitis, can cause serious neurological damage and even death.

Intervertebral disc

Intervertebral discs (IVDs) are the soft gel-like structures that sit between our vertebrae. The primary functions of the disc are to allow movement between vertebral bodies and to transfer weight from one vertebral body to the next. The disc creates a space between the vertebral bodies—thus

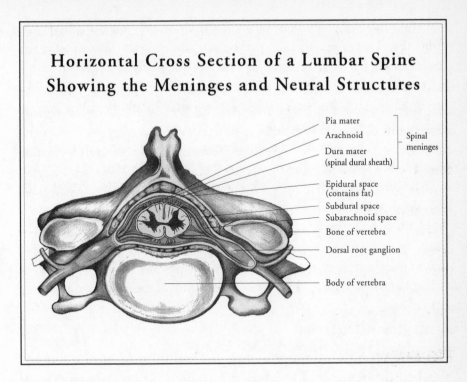

Horizontal Cross Section of a Lumbar Spine Showing the Meninges and Neural Structures

Pia mater
Arachnoid ⎤ Spinal
Dura mater ⎦ meninges
(spinal dural sheath)

Epidural space
(contains fat)
Subdural space
Subarachnoid space
Bone of vertebra

Dorsal root ganglion

Body of vertebra

permitting the upper vertebra to tilt forwards and backwards without hitting the vertebrae above or beneath it.

The intervertebral disc has two major parts. There is a central 'ball bearing' part which is made up of a jelly-like substance called the nucleus pulposus. This part transfers loads from one disc to the next and allows movement between vertebrae. The second part of the disc is called the annulus fibrosis, which consists of several concentric rings which contain the nucleus in a central position. The nuclear material is toxic to the body if it escapes from the disc and can cause an inflammatory reaction resulting in pain.

Then there are fibrous concentric rings called lamellae that prevent the jelly-like matter from entering the rest of the body.

With age, the intervertebral discs slowly dehydrate to approximately 70 per cent by the age of 60. Optimally, the intervertebral disc resists spinal compression while permitting limited movements. Together, the nucleus and annulus distribute loads across the vertebral bodies even when the spine is bent, flexed or extended. A third component of the disc is the vertebral endplate. Each disc has two endplates, which are layers of cartilage that cover the top and bottom aspects of each disc.

Pain-sensitive nerve fibres normally penetrate only the outermost part of the disc. Therefore, you only experience pain from the disc if you injure its outermost part. Certain injuries can permanently alter the structure and function of a disc. However, this does not mean that the disc will be forever painful. In this book we will explore rehabilitation options that are open to sufferers of such injuries.

Discs are thickest in the lumbar region as they are required to bear greater loads, and are thinnest in the upper thoracic region.

Intervertebral discs are the largest structures in the human body that have no direct blood supply. Nutrients are transported into the disc via blood diffused into the disc from the vertebrae above and below. The pumping of blood occurs thanks to movement of the spine. Conversely, recurrent unloading of the spine allows waste products from the disc to be sucked back into the vertebral body to return to blood circulation.

Annulus fibrosus

The annulus fibrosus is the outer part of the disc, making up approximately half the diameter of the disc. It is comprised of concentric rings of fibrocartilage called lamellae that do not fully encircle the nucleus.

The posterolateral area of the annulus contains the greatest number of incomplete layers. This is one reason discs in the lumbar spine usually tear in the posterolateral region. These factors make the disc thicker in the front and sides, creating a thinner and slightly weaker back portion of the annulus, predisposing it to degenerative change and trauma. Increased **collagen** fibres are found in the outer lamellae, providing extra strength in torsion, **flexion**, **extension** and **lateral flexion** movements. This is helpful because more stress falls on the outer lamellae.

Nucleus pulposus

The nucleus pulposus is the inner part of the disc and comprises about half of the disc diameter. It consists of a water gel held together loosely by a network of fibres. The nucleus attracts and retains water, needed to resist spinal compression. In a newborn baby the fluid content of the nucleus accounts for approximately 90 per cent of the weight, while for a 77-year-old it only accounts for 65 per cent of the weight.

Diagram of the Annulus Fibrosus Indicating the Angulation of the Collagen Fibres

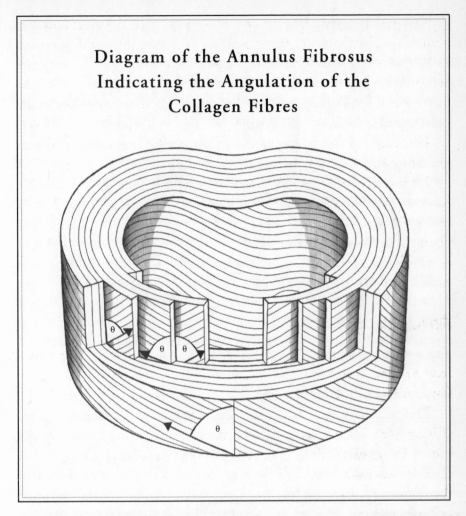

Being a semifluid gel, the nucleus can be deformed under pressure without a reduction in volume. Compression of the nucleus causes it to deform and transmit the applied pressure to its surrounding structures—namely, the annulus fibrosus and vertebral endplates. What occurs can be compared to the effect you get if you have a balloon filled with water and you apply pressure to the balloon. The balloon will deform as the pressure inside the balloon rises and stretches the walls of the balloon in all directions. Although disc problems are a common cause of back pain, the nucleus lacks a nerve supply, and thus cannot by itself be the primary source of back pain. The pain in disc sufferers originates in other structures that are compromised by the failure of the nucleus.

Vertebral endplates

Vertebral endplates are thin layers of cartilage about 0.6 to 1 mm thick that cover the top and bottom of the disc.

Vertebral endplates are responsible for the growth in height of the vertebral bodies and prevent the nucleus from bulging into the vertebral body.

When we are born our endplates have many small blood vessels; however, these blood vessels gradually die off during the first 10–15 years of life, leaving small, weakened areas which make the vertebral body more susceptible to intravertebral disc prolapses called Schmorl's nodes. These can be seen on X-rays, CT and MRI. They weaken the endplate and may be a precursor to collapse of the endplate and/or disc degeneration.

As mentioned previously, discs do not have a direct blood supply. They depend on the nutrients supplied by the adjacent vertebral bodies, which exchange nutrients and waste products via the endplates by means of diffusion. Endplate permeability decreases with ageing, resulting in diminished transport of nutrients and waste products.

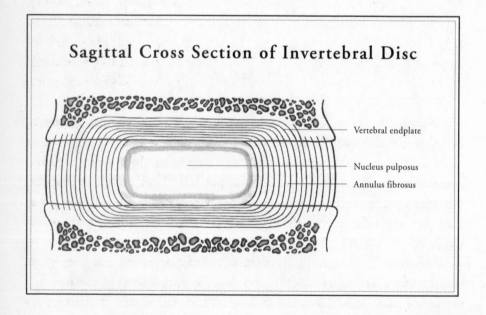

Sagittal Cross Section of Invertebral Disc

Vertebral endplate

Nucleus pulposus

Annulus fibrosus

Disc nerve supply

The inner one-third of the disc has no nerve supply. Only the outer one-third, and rarely the outer two-thirds, of the disc has nerves. Therefore, injury or damage to the inner third of the disc goes unnoticed. Injury to the outer third part of the disc will result in what is termed 'discogenic pain'. Typically in the lumbar spine this causes generalised referred low back pain and possible buttock and thigh pain that can extend to the knee. The posterior aspect of the disc is innervated by the sinuvertebral nerve. This nerve is involved in most cases of back pain. One therapy, which we'll discuss later in this book, involves cutting the sinuvertebral nerve.

Facet joints

Facet joints connect adjacent vertebrae together. Each vertebra (except for the top two) has two facet joints—one on the left and one on the right; however, anatomical variations can occur between individuals. Lumbar facet joints contain a joint space, membrane, cartilage surfaces and a fibrous capsule.

There are several structures within the **joint capsule**. During spinal flexion, the facet joints glide upward some 5 mm to 8 mm, thus exposing the joint cartilage of the facet joint. A tissue pad is understood to act as a protective feature of the facet joint when the cartilage is exposed. There are two 'mini-discs' or menisci per facet joint, which are small discs that sit in between the two articular processes. The purpose of these discs is to lubricate the joint.

The lumbar and sacral multifidii muscles insert or attach into the fibrous capsules. It is believed that the muscle protects the capsule from being caught inside the joint during movements.

The facet joints help movements, resist force and bear weight. As we age the intervertebral discs become narrower, which leads to greater weight bearing on the facet joints. Facet joints are not designed to withstand great loads and it is believed that the extra compression leads to degeneration of the joints.

Regardless of exercise, facet joints naturally degenerate with age. By the age of 60 to 69 years, 89 per cent of the population have facet joint osteoarthrosis. The L4/5 and L5/S1 joints are the most commonly affected. Having facet joint osteoarthrosis is not always associated with low back pain.

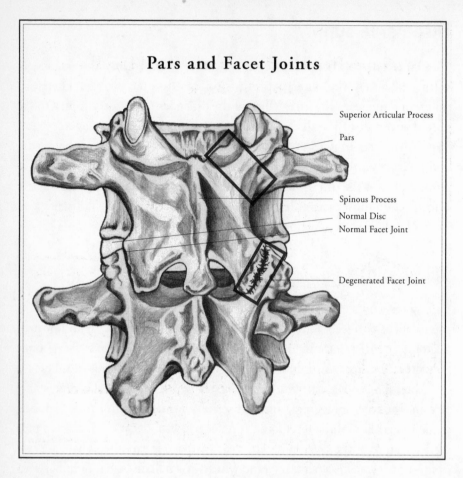

Pars and Facet Joints

Superior Articular Process

Pars

Spinous Process
Normal Disc
Normal Facet Joint

Degenerated Facet Joint

Facet joints are covered in a thin layer of cartilage that is strongly held together by a joint capsule (a ligament-like structure that encircles the joint). The capsule has many small nerve endings that are sensitive to movement and pain; these are often reported as a source of low back pain. The good news is that by treating one facet joint you can affect the vertebral segment above and below it as well because they all have the same nerve supply.

Muscles

There are three major types of muscle found in the human body—skeletal, cardiac and smooth muscle. Cardiac muscle is only found in the heart, while smooth muscle is found in arteries, lymph tissue and various organs

Superficial and Intermediate Muscles of the Back

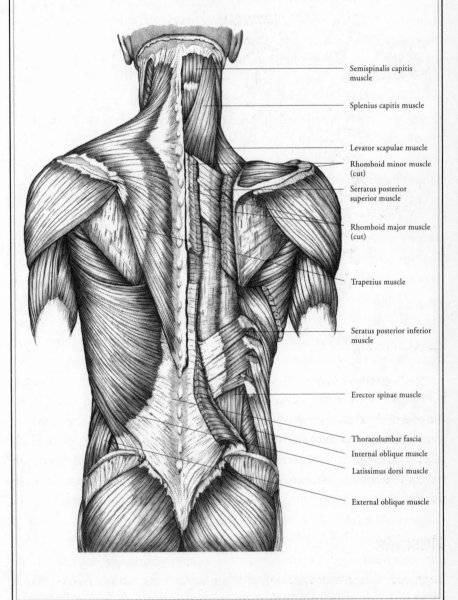

Semispinalis capitis muscle

Splenius capitis muscle

Levator scapulae muscle

Rhomboid minor muscle (cut)

Serratus posterior superior muscle

Rhomboid major muscle (cut)

Trapezius muscle

Serratus posterior inferior muscle

Erector spinae muscle

Thoracolumbar fascia

Internal oblique muscle

Latissimus dorsi muscle

External oblique muscle

such as the intestines. The type we are interested in here is called skeletal muscle. Skeletal muscle is under voluntary control, which is good news to those suffering back pain. Skeletal muscle is what we are referring to when we speak of the muscles of the back.

There are several layers of muscles in the back (see diagram). As a general rule the more superficial muscles (top layer) are movers, while the deepest muscles tend to be stabilisers. Some muscles have dual roles as a mover and a stabiliser. The simplistic view that a single muscle is the sole cause of back pain is outdated. Current understanding of human musculoskeletal function and physiology indicates that the most common scenario of back pain involving muscles includes several muscles which contribute to the overall condition in varying degrees. This is good news for those who suffer from back pain, because working on muscle strength and balance is something we can all do. The exercises outlined in this book are a great place to start.

Back muscles are seldom the primary cause of back pain; muscles tend to react to some other primary cause of back pain. People suffering from an acute intervertebral disc protrusion will often have accompanying **antalgia** (lateral shift of the body to one side), where they avoid aggravating the injured disc. The body will involuntarily contract specific muscles to cause this lean. If you try to work against the lean, you will experience pain. The problem is not the muscles, they are simply trying to protect you from your activity. Having muscle treatment on these guarding muscles may provide temporary relief or an improved range of motion. However, it does not address the cause of the muscle guarding, which may be the intervertebral disc, and therefore will not provide long-term relief.

It has been confirmed that back muscles can be a source of back pain. What is debatable is the actual cause of the muscle pain, which is alleged to come from sprain/strain, spasm, imbalance and trigger points.

Muscle spasms are thought to occur due to some postural abnormality or flow-on effect to joint pain, where muscles become chronically contracted and therefore painful. If this is correct, the only plausible mechanism for the generation of pain is from lack of blood flow, but more research in this area needs to confirm this idea. It is unclear whether muscle spasm is due to contraction or **hyperreflexia**. Further research needs to be carried out before the notion of muscle spasm is accepted.

It is believed that muscle imbalances can lead to back pain. For every muscle in the body that creates movement, there is a complementary muscle that does the opposite movement. Imbalances are thought to occur between these complementary muscles. Be aware that currently there is no concrete evidence to prove this theory.

It is our view that muscle imbalances do cause back pain, although it happens indirectly. For further discussion, see Liebenson in References. The muscular system is controlled by two major systems of the body: the central nervous system and the musculoskeletal system. Dysfunction in either of these two systems can result in changes in the muscular system, such as altered muscle tone, muscle contraction, muscle balance, coordination and performance.

Muscles tend to develop weakness or tightness not in a random fashion but rather in predictable muscle imbalance patterns. The development of these patterns can be predicted clinically and preventative measures should be taken because these patterns can spread to involve the entire muscular system. Muscle tone can and ought to be assessed to properly treat muscles. Muscle tension should not be considered an isolated tissue response (that is, a single muscle involvement), but rather as a systemic myofascial (multiple muscles and soft tissue involvement) response.

Muscle imbalances usually precede muscle pain, so it is important to identify these imbalances before the muscles become painful.

Muscles don't actually attach to bones

All bones are covered by a thin fibrous membrane called **periosteum**. The function of the periosteum is to provide a point of attachment for muscles and ligaments as well as provide nourishment to the bone through the blood vessels and nerves contained within it. Despite what many people believe and what most anatomy books show, muscles do not actually attach to bone. They attach to the periosteum surrounding the bone. This has huge biomechanical and anatomical implications because direct connections can be observed between structures at opposing ends of the body. For instance, tension in your right foot can cause tightness in the right side of the neck. Thomas Myers, author of *Anatomy Trains*, termed these connections 'myofascial meridians'. He highlighted the existence of 12 or so major myofascial lines in the body, which govern the function and posture of the body. For more information visit www.anatomytrains.com.

Fascia

Fascia is the Latin word for band or bandage. Fascia surrounds and connects every muscle, even the tiniest muscle cell, and every single organ of the body. Fascia is a dense, connective tissue that surrounds muscles, groups of muscles, blood vessels, organs, and nerves; it can be likened to cling wrap around a sandwich. It has elastic properties, blood supply, nerves and contractibility. There are several layers of fascia in the body: superficial fascia, deep fascia and visceral fascia; these layers extend uninterrupted from the head to the toes. Fascia is elastic, allowing it to resist oppositional forces.

Compared to other areas of the musculoskeletal system, fascia has had little scientific attention. We are only beginning to understand fascia, because previously researchers thought fascia had no function and that it was inconsequential residue that was less important than the tissues with which it was associated. What new research is bringing to light is the fact that fascia plays a major role in how our body functions.

Fascia has many functions, which include creating separate compartments for muscles, being a soft tissue skeleton for muscle attachments, encouraging oxygenated blood supply in the lower limbs, dissipating stress or strain at bone ends and protecting underlying structures.

Recent research has demonstrated that fascia may be able to actively contract in a smooth muscle-like manner and thus can influence musculoskeletal biomechanics. Specialised connective tissue cells (myofibroblasts), have been proven to actively contract and relax when stimulated. Examples of fascia actively contracting include wound healing and in pathological fascial contractures like Dupuytren's contracture (bent finger tendon) and frozen shoulder. The middle section of the back has the highest density of myofibroblasts of any fascia in the human body. There is also a correlation between the level of physical activity and myofibroblast density. Myofibroblast density can vary greatly between different people.

How fascia can bring pain relief to back pain sufferers is due to their responsiveness to manual pressure.

Fascia has recently been identified as the largest sensory organ of the human body.

Sacroiliac joints

The sacroiliac joint is the junction between the sacrum and the ilium bone. There are two of these joints in the body, one on either side of the sacrum. They are important because they effectively connect the torso to the lower limbs. They allow one side of the hip and the pelvis to flex while the other hip and pelvis are in extension. The articular portion of the ilium and sacrum are covered by a thick layer of cartilage, which provides a smooth surface for the bone to move. The sacroiliac joints only move

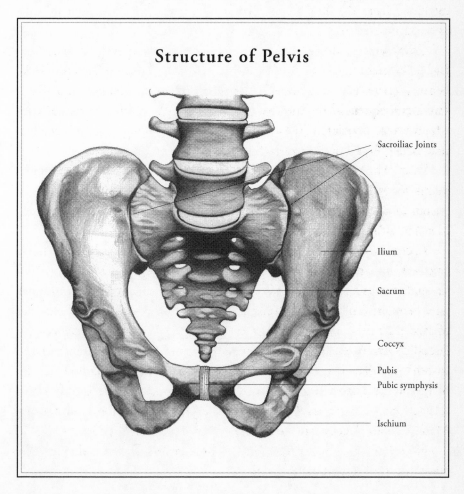

Structure of Pelvis

Sacroiliac Joints

Ilium

Sacrum

Coccyx

Pubis
Pubic symphysis

Ischium

about 1–3 degrees; however, the movement is essential for proper bio-mechanical function of the spine. The sacrum and ilium are held together by several thick and very strong ligaments: the two main ones are the posterior sacroiliac ligament (back) and the anterior sacroiliac ligament (front).

My back pain story
Drew Ginn

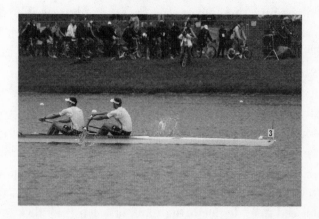

By the time he was 25 years old, Drew Ginn had already won two World Championships and a gold medal at the Olympics. In 1999 Drew was training for the 2000 Sydney Olympics when disaster struck. While he was doing squats at the gym, Drew felt a sudden excruciating pain in his low back and he immediately sought medical attention. MRI scans showed that Drew had ruptured his L4–L5 disc, which was now compressing his left L5 nerve root, causing severe pain, numbness and weakness in his left thigh and leg. Drew required treatment from various practitioners several times per week, just so he could train each day. Eventually after a year of this routine, the stress of rigorous training took its toll on Drew's back. Treatments such as physiotherapy, myofascial work and acupuncture were no longer relieving his back pain. It was at this point that Drew consulted again with his orthopaedic surgeon. The surgeon had been reluctant to perform surgery in the beginning, but now came to the conclusion that back surgery was the only viable option. The surgery was successful; they were able to remove the part of the disc that was compressing Drew's spinal nerve, which immediately alleviated his excruciating thigh and leg pain. Drew was forced to miss his home Olympic Games in Sydney 2000 while he recovered from surgery. Following the surgery, his surgeon told Drew he should never row again, as he was at risk of doing further damage to his back. He decided to take this on as a challenge rather than a problem.

Although he had some of the best specialists in Australia work on him, he felt disenchanted by the whole experience, feeling as though they treated him more like a problem than a person.

Drew embarked on the arduous and time-consuming task of rehabilitation, a daily regime that meant after over a year he was able to return to a level where he could again compete in rowing at the highest level. Due to some of the irreversible effects of the back issue, Drew was forced to re-evaluate how he trained and competed. Drew had to modify his stroke so as to not overload his back, which could have led to further damage; he also radically changed his training methods. He no longer lifted weights, which he found caused him to tighten up. He began to experiment with functional movements and core-stability by incorporating certain aspects of yoga, pilates and aikido to increase his range of motion and keep him limber. Drew and a few of his teammates began attending yoga classes and they noticed that, despite being super fit, their flexibility and range of motion was poor compared to those yoga clients who weren't professional athletes. Drew found he was better able to deal with the repeat movement of rowing after yoga exercise, even though the exercises themselves didn't involve rowing movement.

Drew went on to win the World Championships in 2003, and captured the gold medal in the coxless pair at the 2004 Athens Olympics. However, during the 2008 Olympics his low back reared its ugly head again. During a heat of the men's coxless pair, Drew felt something 'go' in his low back. In spite of debilitating low back pain, Drew rowed the Olympic final and won his third Olympic gold medal from three Olympics. A few weeks later he returned to Australia and could barely walk due to numbness and weakness in his right foot. Scans revealed that Drew had the injury reoccur at the same L4–L5 disc position. This time it was on the right side, which was now causing him excruciating thigh and leg pain, numbness and foot drop (inability to bend the ankle). Two days after returning from the Olympics, Drew was having a second back surgical procedure. Drew was again told by his surgeon that he should retire from rowing or risk further back problems. Drew heeded the advice this time, but slowly and methodically went about the task of rehabilitating his back. In the beginning Drew simply wanted to be able to perform activities of daily living. It wasn't until a few months into his rehabilitation that the thought of rowing entered his mind.

Drew competed in his fourth Olympics in London and won the silver medal in the men's coxless four. In his words:

'Earlier in my career when I got injured, therapists would isolate the area they were going to work on and say, "We need to rebuild that up and then we need to get you stronger".

'What I found was that for me this approach almost made things worse, because I would continually fall into the same injury cycle . . . what I do now is to do handstands, handsprings, jumping on one foot, running backward, which not only creates awareness, but also allows the body to figure out what to do with the right sort of intention.'

The take-home message of this story is never give up or accept doctors' points of view as the only interpretation of the facts. There are many options available on the subject of back pain, so keep trying until you find one that works for you consistently.

2 Causes of back pain

It is important to appreciate the many possible causes or sources of back pain. Back pain may be due to either mechanical causes (sometimes called 'simple back pain'), or more rarely to a disease or pathological process. The good news is that less than 2 per cent of cases of low back pain are due to serious disease processes.

In working out the cause of low back pain, first practitioners must establish whether the back pain is mechanical or pathological. To determine this, indicators of pathology are assessed. We call these indicators 'red flags'. If a patient has more than one of these red flags in their background history, this mandates the use of diagnostic procedures such as medical imaging (X-ray, CT scan, MRI scan), blood test or other special examinations or tests to identify whether or not a pathology is present. If not present, a mechanical cause for the back pain is investigated. A list of commonly accepted red flag indicators is presented below.

Pathological causes of back pain

Here is a list of some of the more common pathological causes of back pain. In no way is this list complete, but it does provide insight into the wide range of possible causes of back pain.

- **Infections:** back pain can be a symptom of various infections, be it viral or bacterial in origin. Examples of bacterial infections include bone infection (osteomyelitis) and meningitis (infection of the meninges which envelop the spinal cord). Shingles is an example of a viral infection that can cause back pain. Flu symptoms also commonly involve back pain.

- **Neoplasms:** these are malignant or benign tumours. Examples of benign tumours that may cause back pain include spinal meningiomas and neurofibromas. Examples of malignant tumours that may cause back pain include myelomas and lymphomas.
- **Organ problems:** several organs refer pain to the back, thus diseases of these organs will result in referral pain in the back. Kidney disorders cause flank pain, which is pain in the back near the base of the ribs.
- **Specific diseases**
  - **Ankylosing spondylitis:** this is a chronic systemic inflammatory disorder affecting the spine as well as other joints of the body. The sacroiliac joints are commonly affected and can cause the joints and ligaments of the spine to be replaced by solid bone. Currently no cure is available; however, genetic and auto-immune factors are believed to be implicated.
  - **Scheuermann's disease:** this disease affects the vertebral end plates. It tends to occur mainly in the thoracic spine (middle spine) and causes excessive kyphotic curvature of the spine, reducing normal spinal movement.
  - **Paget's disease:** this is a chronic bone-remodelling disorder that results in enlarged and misshapen bones. The disease may involve virtually any bone in the human body. It mainly affects adults over the age of 55, and men are twice as likely to be sufferers. The disease is often treated with bisphosphonate drugs, but currently there is no cure.
  - **Diffuse Idiopathic Skeletal Hyperostosis (DISH):** DISH is a form of non-inflammatory spine arthritis, whereby calcium is deposited in parts of the vertebrae. It may or may not cause pain, but restricted spinal movement is more prevalent. DISH tends to occur in men over 50 years of age and those with a predisposition to heart disease, high blood pressure, obesity and stroke. The cause of DISH is not known.
  - **Atherosclerosis:** hardening of the arteries may be a source of back pain in some individuals. Complications of atherosclerosis, such as an abdominal aortic aneurysm, can cause fluctuating low back pain in some individuals.

Pathological conditions causing low back pain and their indicators (red flags)

Indicators for cancer	Prior history of cancer Unexplained weight loss Aged over 50 years Aged under 17 years old Night pain
Indicators for infection	Persistent fever (temperature over 38°C) Recent bacterial infection Night pain History of intravenous drug abuse Lumbar spine surgery within the last year Recent wound in spine region or elsewhere
Immune system compromise	Long-term corticosteroid drug use Organ transplant HIV (human immunodeficiency virus) Diabetes
Indicators for cauda equina syndrome	Loss of bladder control Loss of bowel control Progressive weakness or numbness in the legs Pins and needles sensation or numbness in the saddle area Loss of sensation in the legs
Indicators for vertebral fracture	Long-term corticosteroid drug use Age greater than 70 years History of osteoporosis or other bone-weakening disease Any physical trauma over the age of 50 Recent major injury Severe spinal tenderness Very limited spinal movement
Indicators for aortic aneurysm	Pulsating mass in the abdomen High blood pressure Age greater than 60 years Pain while resting Night pain
Other	No improvement with treatment over six weeks Back pain unrelated to movement Abnormal response to treatment

Mechanical causes of back pain

Here is a list of some of the most common mechanical causes of low back pain. Mechanical essentially means non-pathological. Mechanical causes are the major reason that people experience low back pain. These causes include the following:

- Annular tear of the disc
- Coccydynia
- Disc protrusion/herniation
- Disc lesion with radiculopathy
- Facet joint syndrome
- Failed back surgery syndrome
- Acute locked back
- Hypermobility and hypermobility syndrome
- Internal disc disruption/derangement
- Lumbar instability
- Muscle injuries
- Myofascial trigger points
- Nerve entrapment
- Sacroiliac joint dysfunction
- Spinal stenosis
- Spondylolysis/spondylolisthesis
- Vertebral endplate fracture
- Vertebral compression fracture
- Multiple causes of back pain

The following two lists show the most common causes of both acute and chronic back pain.

Disc injuries

Intervertebral discs slowly degenerate with age. This is a natural process that begins as early as 15 years of age. The rate at which a disc degenerates varies from person to person, and is dependent on the disc position in the spine. Lower discs (lumbar) have greater loads placed on them and they tend to degenerate more quickly than discs further up the spine. With age, the disc becomes less sponge-like and retain less water.

Causes of *acute* non-specific mechanical back pain

Cause	Percentage
Facet joints	10%
Sacroiliac joint	10%
Unknown origin	50–60%
Disc without sciatica	10–20%
Disc with sciatica	10%

Source: Estimates from personal communication with C. Liebenson

Causes of *chronic* non-specific mechanical back pain

Cause	Percentage
Internal disc disruption	39%
Facet joints	15%
Sacroiliac joint	12%
Unknown origin	34%

Sources: McGill, Liebenson

Approximately 80 per cent of all lumbar disc injuries occur in the bottom two lumbar discs (L4–5 and L5–S1), which usually degenerate quicker than the other lumbar discs. In the cervical spine a similar process occurs, with the C5–C6 and C6–C7 discs degenerating faster than the rest of the cervical spine. Thoracic disc injuries are quite rare compared to cervical and lumbar disc injuries; however, they do occur.

Disc injuries differ from normal age-related degeneration. Degeneration is a normal process that occurs in every spine with age, while disc injuries do not occur in everyone.

Annular height loss in bulging discs can lead to more than 50 per cent of the compressive load on the lumbar spine being resisted by the facet joints instead of the discs (not a desired outcome).

With increasing age, the nucleus tends to bulge vertically into the vertebral bodies. The result is less pressure on the nucleus and more pressure on the annulus, causing the annulus to bulge outward and some-times inward. Changes in pressure on the disc result in a marked loss of structure. In effect, the disc behaves like a flat tyre. Once a disc is injured or damaged it will never fully heal; however, this does not imply that an injured disc will always be a painful disc. Many people go on to live pain-free lives after a disc injury.

Damaged discs react to weight bearing in a haphazard manner. Their shock-absorbing function can become reduced or disappear.

Learn the loads

The intervertebral discs have different loads placed on them based on your body posture/position. This has major implications on the biomechanics and physiology of the spine. The most unloaded position for the lumbar discs is lying flat on your back, while the most loaded position is sitting slouched. It is important to know and understand these loads in order to protect your back from stressful or damaging loads. Certain postures place less load on the spine, which can help relieve back pain as well as reduce spinal wear and tear. Sitting actually places greater load on the discs than lying down or standing. This does not imply that it is always best to stand or lie down; certain back conditions are most comfortable in the seated position. A general rule to follow is 'if it hurts, don't do it'. So if it hurts to stand upright and feels better to sit, by all means have a seat.

Annular tear of the disc

Since the inner two-thirds of the annulus is not supplied with nerve fibres, the outer third is the only part of the disc which can generate pain.

To be clear, an annular tear is not the same as a herniated or bulging disc. For a bulging disc to occur, fibres from the innermost annular layers must be torn, allowing the central nuclear material to move to the edge. The remaining outermost layers attempt to retain the nuclear material within the disc, causing substantial strain on the outer layers, which begin to creep. This leads to the appearance of a bulge in the **posterior** or poste-rolateral aspect of the disc.

In the case of a disc protrusion, the nucleus seeps across several layers of the annulus to reach the outer third of the disc, which causes back pain. In the case of a herniated disc, the nucleus escapes the disc to reach the spinal canal where it can irritate or compress the spinal nerves.

Annular tears are often broken into three categories:

- **Peripheral or rim lesion:** this form of injury is defined as discrete tears of the outer layers of the annulus fibrosus, parallel and adjacent to one or both end-plates. They are frequently accompanied by in-growth of vascular granulation tissue, sometimes extending into the middle layers of the annulus. Also associated with rim lesions is **osteophyte** formation and/or adjacent bone marrow may be replaced by granulation tissue.
- **Circumferential lesion:** this is the most common form of annular tear found in the **anterior** and posterior annulus. These lesions sometimes display vascular in-growth and cystic degeneration, and are commonly seen in relation to rim lesions.
- **Radial lesion:** this form of lesion tends to be found in patients with advanced disc degeneration. Clefts form parallel to or at oblique angles to the vertebral end-plate, and radiate out from the nucleus pulposus to the outer lamellae of the annulus.

Presentation

An annular tear can occur without cause or after a specific traumatic event. They can be asymptomatic, in which case the patient is unaware of when or how the tear occurred. With symptomatic presentations, pain can be sharp with specific movements such as **flexion** or **rotation** to one side; otherwise, it can present as a generalised constant dull ache in the low back area. There may be pain referral into the buttocks and back of the thigh, but pain generally does not go below the knee unless there is nerve root involvement. Hard neurological signs or symptoms such as pins and needles, numbness or weakness are absent. If neurological signs or symptoms are present, a diagnosis of a simple annular tear cannot be made.

Causes

Annular tears are due to repeated, forced end-range rotation of the intervertebral joint. Over time the annulus layers break, just as a repeatedly flexed piece of metal will fatigue and fracture. The addition of spinal flexion with rotation further increases the risk of injury, especially at the vulnerable rear of the annulus.

Diagnosis

Annular tears are difficult to definitively diagnose due to the fact that they are not visible in medical imaging such as CT scans or X-rays. However, annular tears can be visualised using special techniques. One method is to inject the nucleus pulposus with a contrast medium as well as a local anaesthetic. If the disc is the true source of pain, the local anaesthetic will relieve the pain, and the contrast medium will outline the tear, which can be seen on a CT scan as a crescent in the outer annulus fibrosus. This procedure is still experimental and there are no studies to validate its effectiveness as yet.

Treatment

Increasing the pressure on the disc will generally make the back pain worse, so try to minimise prolonged sitting, and repetitive bending or twisting. Standing decreases pressure on the injured disc and often helps to relieve low back pain associated with annular tears. Most tears will self repair with time. A scar tissue plug normally forms in the outer layers of the tear, thereby blocking any potential leaks. Unfortunately the plug does not form across all the layers of the annulus, to protect the disc from future tears.

Disc herniation

A disc herniation is defined as a localised displacement of disc material beyond the limits of the intervertebral disc space. The disc material may be nucleus, cartilage, fragmented apophyseal bone, annular tissue or any combination of these parts.

Natural history of a herniated disc shows clinical symptoms tend to disappear in up to 50 per cent of patients, and the herniation can be seen to shrink on CT scans or MRI scans within nine months after the onset of back pain. The problem is that most patients aren't willing to hold out that long due to the debilitating pain associated with the disc herniation.

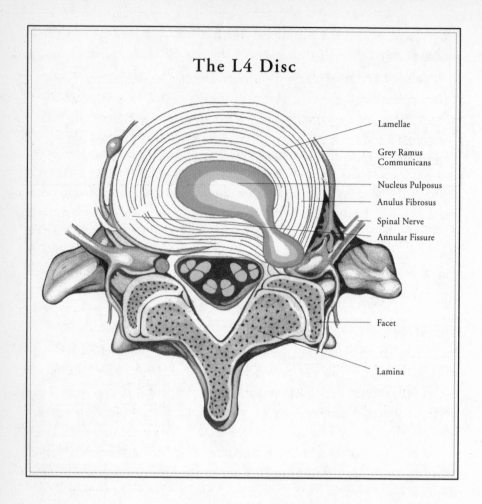

The L4 Disc

Lamellae

Grey Ramus
Communicans

Nucleus Pulposus

Anulus Fibrosus

Spinal Nerve

Annular Fissure

Facet

Lamina

A disc herniation can have associated low back pain or leg pain or both, which can extend below the knee. There is often a long-standing history of low back problems that subsequently resolved. There may be neurological symptoms such as thigh/leg/foot paraesthesia (pins and needles), numbness, burning or weakness.

Disc herniations seem to follow an order of aggravation that begins with pain, progresses to paraesthesia (pins and needles), and finally ends with numbness. Thus, someone who presents with foot numbness due to a disc herniation is in much worse condition than someone with leg pain due to a disc herniation. Also, how far down the leg the symptoms present is an indicator of severity. If a disc patient's leg numbness begins in the calf then a week later progresses to the foot, this indicates a worsening of the

> **Alert**
>
> If you get any unexplained bowel or bladder incontinence (partial or total loss of bowel or bladder control) or saddle area numbness, go immediately to the emergency department of the nearest hospital. These symptoms can occur with back pain and may be related to serious spinal nerve damage.

condition. If, however, the reverse occurs and the patient's numbness starts in the calf then regresses to the hamstring, this is seen as an indicator of improvement in the condition.

They didn't even know they had a disc bulge!

A study examined the spines of 98 persons aged between 20 to 80 years who had no history of low back pain. MRI scans of their lumbar spines were carried out and later examined by experienced neuroradiologists. The results demonstrated that 64 per cent of these asymptomatic subjects had at least one intervertebral disc anomaly (disc bulge or protrusion). This tells us that not all disc anomalies picked up on MRIs cause low back pain. The problem is that MRI results are so persuasive that many healthcare practitioners blame disc anomalies as the source of back pain simply due to their presence on a scan.

Disc lesion with radiculopathy

Presentation

The patient often has a past history of low back problems. Pain tends to be relatively constant, which can worsen with either **flexion** or extension of the spine, and is generally moderate to severe in intensity. Pain may develop in the low back region as well as the back of the leg below the knee. Some disc patients present with sharp posterior leg pain or **radiculopathy** below the knee, without any associated back pain. The onset of symptoms is usually sudden after performing a fairly simple bending or twisting movement of the low back. Symptoms are usually worse in the first hour after a person wakes up and then the symptoms settle. Disc lesions can occur at any age but the most common age affected is the 25–35 age group. This is because, as we get older, our discs start to harden and become less likely to seep out or herniate.

Causes

There are two theories to explain nerve-related leg pain due to a disc lesion. The first is that the nucleus creates a bulge or herniation which directly compresses the nerves that exit the spine. The second is that the nucleus releases chemicals which irritate the nerves or causes an inflammatory reaction.

Diagnosis

Due to the fact that 80 per cent of all lumbar disc lesions occur at L4–L5 or L5–S1 levels, practitioners typically focus on these areas. Disc lesions do not appear on standard X-rays, thus X-rays are of little use for the diagnosis of a disc lesion. MRI is currently the gold standard for imaging a disc lesion; however, CT scans also show disc lesions, but exposes the patient to some radiation. The CT image is also of a poorer quality than MRI.

Treatment

Manual treatment continues to be a main non-invasive treatment approach with disc lesions. Spinal manipulation has been shown to be effective in providing short-term pain relief in the early stages of disc lesions, but not for long-term relief. There is some controversy regarding whether side-posture manipulation is appropriate for disc lesions. If the rotary component of the adjustment is minimised and the patient is pre-tested with mild mobilisation at the segment to be adjusted, cautious side-posture adjusting is a possible alternative. Other non-rotary manual treatment approaches exist, such as flexion-distraction spinal blocking. Rotation movements during exercises, spinal mobilisation or manipulation are best avoided.

Although a last resort, the short-term success rate after surgery for lumbosacral disc herniation is around 95 to 98 per cent with a 2 to 6 per cent incidence of true recurrence of herniation. The rate of success

> *Alert*
>
> Lying down for long periods causes the discs to fill up with water (swell), which in turn creates more pressure within the disc and can result in more pain. Furthermore, prolonged bed rest has been shown to lead to wasting of low back muscles. Therefore, you should be mindful to avoid prolonged bed rest other than sleeping. During rest you should get up and move around for at least five minutes every hour.

drops down to 80 per cent for the long term due to symptoms associated with failed back surgery syndrome.

Recommendations

Each patient with these disc issues is unique and, therefore, necessitates a thorough examination and plan in order to safely and effectively resolve this condition. Figuring out which exercises and activities ought to be prescribed or avoided needs to be well planned and analysed before being adopted by the patient. In relation to activities, a general guideline is to avoid or at least minimise activities that exacerbate symptoms. However, it should be expected that if a patient has poor fitness, some exercise-related discomfort or pain may be unavoidable; this does not mean that the exercises are harmful. It is important for the patient to be able to distinguish hurt versus harm.

Here are some general guidelines if you are unsure what to do. Avoid bending, twisting or lifting when suffering a new pain. Prolonged flexion or end-range movements are generally not recommended. Weight lifting should be avoided until the disc-related symptoms are stabilised. Sit-ups, crunches and reverse sit-ups compress discs and can further exacerbate the condition. Specific core-stability exercises done with a neutral spine are recommended (see spine-sparing core-stability exercises in the colour section). Continuation of normal activities and early return to work protocols have been shown to be helpful. While bed rest may be recommended in the earliest stage of the condition, it has been shown that bed rest of greater than 72 hours can cause negative effects.

There is no such thing as a slipped disc!

Invertebral discs can bulge, protrude, herniate, sequestrate and degenerate, but they do not slip. These terms describe the extent or form of disc injury, which can be only properly diagnosed with a CT scan or MRI. Discs cannot be seen on a plain X-ray, so these conditions cannot be diagnosed this way.

Facet joint syndrome

Facet joint syndrome (lumbar zygapophysial joint arthropathy) affects up to 15 per cent of patients with chronic low back pain. A problem that practitioners encounter is that facet joint pain is difficult to diagnose clinically. Diagnostic blocks (injection of anaesthetic into the facet joint) are the only method currently available to positively diagnose the condition. X-rays, single photon emission computer tomography (SPECT), CT scans and MRIs can demonstrate structural changes of the facet joint. However, these changes are not indicative of pain as these changes occur just as frequently in asymptomatic individuals. Injuries to the facet joint often involve the **joint capsule**. Unfortunately, tears to the facet joint capsule are also undetectable by X-ray, CT or MRI. Nearly 60 per cent of adults show some signs of facet joint degeneration by the age of 30. Degeneration continues to steadily increase until people are in their 60s at which point it becomes unavoidable.

Acute locked back

Presentation

Another common cause of facet joint pain is facet joint **meniscus** extrapment. Onset is usually sudden and generally occurs after a relatively simple movement such as rising from a bent-over position, or misjudging a step when stepping off a curb. Pain is usually well-localised to the low back area with some hip, buttock or posterior thigh referral pain occurring above the knee. The patient often presents in a slightly flexed position in an attempt to avoid pain.

Causes
Due to flexion, the meniscus is drawn out of the joint, and then the meniscus fails to re-enter the joint when the person returns to an upright posture.

Diagnosis
Facet joint problems are often difficult to differentiate from disc or nerve root problems due to the overlapping areas of pain. There are a few distinguishing features of facet joint syndrome such as the absence of neurological symptoms, absence of nerve tension signs, pain that is localised with Kemp's manoeuvre (an orthopaedic test) and referred pain that does not extend below the knee. Currently the condition of meniscus extrapment cannot be reliably detected with medical imaging techniques.

Treatment
Acute locked back tends to respond quickly and favourably to spinal manipulative therapy. The goal of the manipulation is to gap the facet joint, which allows the meniscus to return to its normal position in the joint cavity. Medical treatments include radiofrequency facet denervation and facet joint injections. There is mixed support for facet joint injections in the literature. Facet denervation is a more invasive procedure, but research has shown positive effects for select chronic low back pain sufferers.

Failed back surgery syndrome (FBSS)

Failed back surgery syndrome is non-specific and may not be the best term for this condition, as it implies failure on the part of the surgeon or the patient, when neither may be true. One study found that it was possible to make a specific diagnosis in 94 per cent of patients diagnosed with FBSS. This highlights the need for a more specific diagnosis than FBSS. Causes of FBSS include scar tissue fibrosis and adhesions, spinal instability, recurrent herniated disc and inadequate decompression.

It often takes months or even up to a year for patients to recover from various spinal surgeries, so patients need to be tolerant and diligent with their post-operative rehabilitation. A general rule is that the longer a patient had back pain prior to surgery and the more extensive the surgery required, the longer and more difficult the post-operative rehabilitation will be.

Despite advances in spinal surgical technology the rates of FBSS remain the same. In the United Kingdom there are approximately 2000 new cases of FBSS per year. It is estimated that 5 to 10 per cent of lumbar surgery patients end up with some form of complication resulting in FBSS.

Spinal cord stimulation (SCS) uses an electrical device that is implanted in the body of the patient. The device has leads that connect to the spinal cord. It works by stimulating nerve fibres in the spinal cord, which inhibits the conduction of pain to the brain according to the pain gate theory. SCS is often successful in reducing perceptible pain, but does not eliminate it, as it simply masks the sensation of pain by producing tingling or numbness instead. There are complications that can arise from SCS such as lead migration, lead breakage, infection, haematomas, cerebrospinal fluid (CSF) leak, post-dural puncture headache, discomfort at pulse generator site, seroma and temporary paraplegia. Some of the main benefits of SCS are that patients can reduce taking pain-killers, which can minimise the financial burden and side effects on patients.

Presentation

Patients fail to show any subjective or objective improvement three months after surgery. Failed back surgery syndrome (FBSS) is a syndrome characterised by irreducible pain and various degrees of functional disability following lumbar spine surgery. Failed back surgery syndrome is a diagnosis wherein post-operative symptoms of back or leg pain (or both) persists, including a dull pain in the surgical area and sharp or stabbing pain in the extremities. The pain usually radiates to the hips, buttocks or thighs or all of these.

Causes

The most common cause of FBSS is an incorrect diagnosis of the cause of low back pain prior to surgery. If the lesion operated on was not actually the source of the patient's pain, the results will be poor. In some cases the patient can end up worse than prior to the surgery. Incomplete decompression or a lack of skill or experience on the part of the operating surgeon are also potential causes. Improper or inadequate post-operative rehabilitation are common causes. Choosing a good surgeon is important to minimise the possibility of FBSS. We suggest following the advice in Chapter 5 on how to choose a good therapist.

Diagnosis
FBSS is a diagnosis given to patients post-operatively who have symptoms of persistent back or leg pain, or both, including dull pain in the surgical area and sharp or stabbing pain in the hands and feet. FBSS is not a specific diagnosis but rather is a group heading for various causes of low back pain following surgical intervention. It is therefore advised that a more specific diagnosis be sought in order to treat the condition.

Treatment
Conservative treatment includes chiropractic, physiotherapy and massage therapy. However, if none of these conservative methods produce results, patients can opt for medical treatment such as neuropathic pain medication, minor nerve blocks, transcutaneous electrical nerve stimulation (TENS), anti-inflammatories (**NSAIDs**), intrathecal morphine pump, spinal cord stimulation (SCS) and re-operation. If choosing re-operation, preference may be given to a surgical method that is minimally invasive, which will leave smaller scars and decrease the likelihood of complications. With the many treatment options available it is likely that at least one will be helpful. Concurrently, a careful application of the exercises we recommend in this book may provide superior results.

Hypermobility and hypermobility syndrome

Hypermobility is a term that denotes a joint range of movement that is beyond the normal range. Often individuals with hypermobile joints are referred to as being 'double jointed'. Hypermobility is not a disease, but when pain related to hypermobility ensues, the term 'hypermobility syndrome' (HMS) is given to describe the condition. Unfortunately there is a lack of understanding of HMS in the medical community and the condition often goes undiagnosed or misdiagnosed. Hypermobility in terms of the musculoskeletal system is characterised by loosened connective tissues, muscles and, in particular, ligaments. Hypermobility often affects only a few joints, but some individuals present with multi-joint hypermobility. Specific areas of the body may be more affected than others, and slight asymmetry can be observed. Studies have shown that people with hypermobility have diminished proprioception (position sense), which predisposes them to injury. Over time hypermobility can lead to early joint degeneration due to years of excessive movement.

Presentation

Individuals with hypermobility tend to have decreased muscle tone and strength compared with the general population. More trigger points (see below) are generally found in muscles and ligaments due to the fact that muscles that stabilise joints are often weak and overused. Spinal **scoliosis** occurs more frequently in people with hypermobility. Problems related to hypermobility may not present themselves symptomatically for many years after significant joint or soft tissue damage has led to an injury.

Causes

Hypermobility is estimated to occur in approximately 5 per cent of the population, and is more prevalent in females. Hypermobility is an inherited genetic trait passed on by parents, thus people are born with the condition. Scientists believe it is a variant of Ehlers-Danlos syndrome, also known as 'rubber man disease'. Genes responsible for the production of **collagen** are believed to be involved. Joint hypermobility is also commonly seen in people with Down's syndrome.

Diagnosis

There is no established standard of how much ligamentous laxity equates with hypermobility syndrome. However, the Beighton score and Brighton criteria are two of the most commonly used diagnostic tools for diagnosing hypermobility. To diagnose hypermobility using the Beighton score, a patient must test positive on four or more of a possible nine points of interest, the higher the score the greater the laxity. Check out www.hypermobility.org and search for 'Beighton' and 'Brighton' to see more about the tests.

Treatment

Currently there is no remedy for hypermobility because it is inherited. However, muscle strengthening and sensorimotor exercises have been shown to help. Hypermobility can decrease with age as we naturally lose flexibility, thus children can sometimes grow out of it. Standard conservative treatment includes inactivation of trigger points that cross hypermobile joints—while avoiding extending muscles to their maximum length. Strengthen stabilising muscles around hypermobile joints. Correcting a patient's sense of position can improve stability and muscle reaction time. Because symptomatic problems related to hypermobility may not present for many years, it is prudent to work on stabilising hypermobile joints early on in an attempt to prevent or at least limit its negative effects.

Alert

Treatment that involves stretching techniques is not advised in people with hypermobile joints. This is because stretching lax joints will further destabilise an already loose joint. Holding a posture that is weight-bearing for a prolonged period is also not advised.

Internal disc disruption/derangement

The International Association for the Study of Pain defines internal disc disruption/derangement (IDD) as lumbar pain, with or without referred pain, that stems from an intervertebral disc. Discogenic pain (pain deriving from a disc) is caused by internal disruption of the normal structural and biochemical integrity of the symptomatic disc.

More than a third of all chronic low back pain sufferers have internal disc disruption as the root of their problem. In other words, discogenic pain causes only **referred pain**, not nerve pain (radicular pain) as found with nerve root compression/irritation. Internal disc disruption is not the same a disc degeneration—it is a not a diffuse process affecting the entire disc. Rather, it is a focal disorder affecting a single sector of the annulus fibrosus. Disc degeneration is another matter.

Presentation

Low back and leg pain that does not go below the knee, and not accompanied with pins and needles sensation, numbness or weakness.

Causes

Internal disc disruption is characterised by disruption of the internal architecture of the disc, which becomes painful. However, its external appearance remains unchanged and nerve root compression is not present. Causes include activities that lead to vertebral endplate fractures, which can develop into IDD. These causes include a fall onto the buttocks or the back muscles contracting forcefully, such as when lifting a heavy object or pulling on a stubborn tree root while gardening.

Diagnosis

Currently there is no means available by which IDD can be diagnosed clinically. Standard medical imaging such as myelograms and CT scans will appear normal. In some patients IDD can be detected by MRI. Identification of vertebral endplate abnormalities on MRI have shown high predictive values for discogenic pain. When vertebral endplate abnormalities are found on MRI scans, in most instances the adjacent discs are painful when provoked. Currently the only effective method of diagnosing IDD is discography. The size of radial fissuring (tearing) correlates strongly with the affected disc being painful on disc stimulation. Thus Grade 1 fissures are typically not painful. Grade 2 fissures may or may not be painful, but 70 per cent of all Grade 3 fissures have been shown to be painful.

Treatment

When the condition is mild it can be treated conservatively (without surgery) and the issue resolves within several weeks. However, when the condition is severe it can be resistant to most conservative treatments.

Complications

IDD is commonly misdiagnosed as a disc herniation or it may be ignored by practitioners as patient exaggeration or a psychological problem. Surgery is not necessary for patients with IDD—in fact, surgery can potentially exacerbate the condition.

Recommendations

Two to three weeks of manual therapy such as mobilisation or manipulation is worth trialling. If no improvement occurs, consider getting an opinion from a spinal surgeon. Physical activity and exercise has been shown to effectively strengthen vertebral bodies, rendering them more resistant to endplate fracture.

Alert

Continued treatment in the face of no objective improvement can be dangerous and costly.

Lumbar instability

This is a lack of stability in a given joint. It is important to highlight the distinctions between instability and hypermobility. People are born with hypermobility, it is a genetic trait and it is systemic, meaning that it occurs throughout the body (although some areas may be more affected than others). By contrast, instability is acquired, it is commonly caused by trauma or pathology; we are not born with instability. The damaged joint is the only unstable joint, although the instability may cause problems in adjacent joints, which often have to compensate for the unstable joint. This can lead to myofascial issues but it's uncommon for the unstable joint to cause adjacent joints to become unstable as well.

Instability is a biomechanical term but sometimes it's used out of context. Instability should not be used as an alternative when no other overt anatomical or pathological diagnosis is available. Since it is a biomechanical term, instability must reveal a biomechanical issue.

Spinal instability is a decrease in the ability of the spine to maintain posture and movement without causing deformity, nerve deficit or pain. Some form of temporary lumbar instability can be found in up to 60 per cent of patients with low back pain.

Although it would seem to involve instability, most spondylolistheses (see later in this chapter) do not involve instability. In fact most individuals with grade 1 or 2 spondylolisthesis actually have decreased segmental range of motion (ROM) compared with the general population. Lumbar segmental instability has been cited as a significant cause of chronic low back pain.

A recent study showed that unstable spines are most vulnerable when in a neutral position with low forces being placed on them.

Diagnosis of lumbar instability remains challenging because accurate detection of abnormal or excessive intersegmental motion with CT scans or MRI scans is tricky.

Presentation

Lumbar instability may or may not be symptomatic. Symptomatic patients usually present with localised central lumbar pain around the unstable joint. Back pain associated with lumbar instability is described (in descending order of frequency) as recurrent, constant, 'catching', 'locking', 'giving way' or accompanied by a feeling of instability. Patients usually experience pain during the movement rather than just at the end of the movement. They sometimes have difficulty straightening from a forward-bent posture and may need to use their hands to help them up. A neurological examination will often find no problem.

Causes

Instability can be caused by several factors including spinal injury, disc degeneration, muscle weakness, or poor neuro-muscular coordination. Some habitual movements (bending and flexing) and some surgical procedures have also been implicated as causes of lumbar instability.

Diagnosis

Currently the only validated method for diagnosing instability is radiological examination. Patients can often abolish or significantly decrease their back pain during provocative movements by activating their deep abdominal muscles. Orthopaedic tests for instability often include the prone lumbar instability test and painful arc.

Treatment

Core stability training. Working on patterns of recruitment and co-contraction of local lumbar muscles. Surgical fixation/fusion, only in extreme cases.

> **Alert**
>
> Spinal manipulation or mobilisation of the unstable vertebral segment may aggravate instability. Similarly, passive or active stretching of the soft-tissue structures surrounding the unstable motion segment also can lead to loss of stability.

Muscle injuries

Muscle injuries of the back are quite common; they usually are due to contusion (bruising), strain or laceration. Contusions are due to compression (crush) forces such as a direct blow in contact sports, while strains are due to tensile (overstretch) forces such as reaching into the back seat of a car when sitting in the front seat. When an external force (coming from outside the body) or internal force (force generated within the body) exceeds a muscle's failure tolerance, soft-tissue failure occurs, such as muscle damage. Muscle damage commonly appears in the form of a muscle strain (pulled muscle), tear due to tension, or a contusion (bruise) from a crush/compression injury. Contusions occur at or immediately adjacent to the area of impact, while muscle strains tend to occur close to the join between the muscle and tendons.

Muscles become strained for one of two reasons: either the muscle has been stretched beyond its limits or it has been forced to contract too strongly. The good news is that muscles tend to heal quite well and quickly due to their good blood supply compared to other soft tissues of the body. An interesting aspect about muscle injuries is that soft tissue treatment can (even years after the injury has occurred) provide substantial and sometimes total restoration of function and elimination of pain. Back muscles and **fascia** are damaged with any form of back surgery—some surgeries cause more damage than others. Surgeons continue to come up with less invasive methods to perform back surgery because research demonstrates that greater muscular damage (during surgery) correlates with poorer post-surgical results.

Muscle strain grading

A grading system was developed to help simplify diagnosis and treatment; practitioners classify muscle strains into three grades based on the severity of the injury.

Beginning from least to most severe they are: Grade 1, 2 and 3.

Grade 1

A Grade 1 or 'mild' strain occurs when a muscle is overstretched. There may or may not be some micro-tearing of muscle fibres. There is normally some degree of pain with or without swelling. Some minor bruising may or may not appear a few days after the injury. The prognosis is very good and most patients fully recover in four to six weeks.

Grade 2

A Grade 2 or 'moderate' strain occurs when a muscle is overstretched and some muscle fibres are torn. Symptoms include moderate pain and swelling. Bruising often occurs and this indicates the rupture of some small blood vessels at the site of injury. Joint movement at the nearest associated joint is often restricted and painful. The prognosis is good, and most patients recover in four to six weeks.

Grade 3

A Grade 3 or 'severe' strain is the most serious of the three strains. There is significant tearing of muscle fibres and, in some cases, the muscle can completely tear or rupture sometimes causing a 'pop' sensation or sound. Symptoms include moderate to severe pain, swelling, tenderness and bruising. Movement is either severely restricted or immovable due to pain. The prognosis is poor as the damage is substantial. Recovery ranges from six to twelve weeks for non-complete tears.

With complete tears, surgical reattachment is the only reparative treatment. Some patients may decide to not have surgery, in which case the muscle will no longer function and will atrophy (shrink). There have been reports of spontaneous reattachment of muscles, but this is not common.

Excessive flexibility not always a good thing

Excessive flexibility or joint mobility is medically termed 'hypermobility'. Hypermobile joints are more prone to injury and trauma.

The good news is that you can do something about it—it's called core-stability training. You can learn to tighten up those unstable joints, just like you would tighten the bolts on a wobbly chair. For the low back, the solution is core-stability exercises (refer to the exercises section for examples of core-stability exercises).

Myofascial trigger points

Another potential source of back pain is from an active myofascial trigger point (sometimes referred to as pressure points). A myofascial trigger point is an intensely tender spot on the skin that is associated with a tight band in the muscle. The spot is tender and can give rise to characteristic referred pain, referred tenderness, motor dysfunction, and autonomic phenomena (such as a muscle twitch response). Trigger points are those really tender areas you feel when someone massages your muscles. When you touch them they feel like a frozen pea under your skin. There are several subgroups of myofascial trigger points: active, associated, attachment, central, key, latent, primary and satellite. These should be distinguished from trigger points arising from skin, ligamentous, periosteal or any other non-muscular tissue.

Trigger points account for a large percentage of all myofascial pain, either directly or indirectly. Janet Travell, MD, studied trigger points and published a two-volume book titled *Myofascial Pain and Dysfunction: The Trigger Point Manual*, which is commonly regarded as the bible on the subject of trigger points. Travell also coined the diagnostic term given to pain derived from myofascial trigger points as 'myofascial pain syndrome'.

Latent trigger points cause pain only when compressed or rubbed across; they can become exacerbated and transition to an **active trigger point**. One interesting study found latent trigger points in 54 per cent of 200 asymptomatic persons, and of these was able to cause referred pain in 25 per cent of them. There are two types of active trigger points. The first produces referred pain during activity but becomes reduced or eliminated through rest. The second and more severe type of active trigger point produces referred pain constantly, even at rest.

A satellite trigger point is a focus of hyperirritability in a muscle or its fascia that became active because the muscle was located within the referred pain zone of another trigger point.

A secondary trigger point is a focus of hyperirritability in a muscle or its fascia that became active because its muscle was overloaded as a helper substituting for, or as an antagonist countering the tautness of, the muscle that contained the primary trigger point.

Getting treated sooner rather than later for trigger points has been shown to give better results. The shorter the delay before treatment starts, the less time is required for treatment, and the likelihood of complete recovery increases.

Presentation

Myofascial trigger points can present with one or several of the following symptoms: muscle weakness, decreased or limited joint range of motion, delayed recovery after activity and decreased muscle endurance, muscle hyper-sensitivity and referred pain patterns. Referred pain occurs somewhere other than its origin and is often described as deep, aching or boring muscle pain.

Causes

Travell breaks down the cause of trigger points into two main categories: direct and indirect. Direct causes include mechanical overload, repetitive usage resulting in fatigue, sudden cooling of fatigued muscles and trauma. Indirect causes include organ disease, metabolic dysfunction, arthropathy, endocrine dysfunction, neuropathy, toxicity, myopathy, emotional distress, infection, nutritional deficiencies and other trigger points that activate secondary or satellite trigger points.

Treatment

Several treatment approaches have been reported to be useful in the management of trigger points. These include Nimmo's ischemic pressure, saline injection, acupuncture, massage, manual therapy and spray-and-stretch techniques. The application of heat or ice has also been shown to be helpful in alleviating trigger points discomfort.

Recommendations

Avoid maintaining prolonged postures, repetitive use of fatigued muscles, and sudden cooling of fatigued muscles (as with sitting in front of a fan or air conditioner after intense exercise).

Nerve entrapment

Nerve entrapment occurs when there is direct pressure on a nerve. The pressure can either result in compression or tension being placed on a nerve. The condition may be asymptomatic or symptomatic. There are several conditions that can result in nerve entrapment. The most common ones include spinal-nerve root entrapment caused by a protruding disc, ligament overgrowth, bony spur formation, narrowing of the spinal-nerve channel and tumours.

There is a myofascial theory suggesting that adhesions form between the nerves and surrounding tissue. When the nerve attempts to glide past the adhesion a resultant tension is placed on the nerve and the nerve begins to stretch. Nerves can only be stretched approximately 15 per cent longer than their resting length before the brain kicks in to protect the nerve by inhibiting any further stretching of the nerve. This is why many people are unable to bend over and touch their toes.

There may be different causes of nerve entrapment depending on which area of the body the affected nerve is located. For example, the ulnar nerve in the arm often becomes entrapped in the cubital tunnel (funny bone area) when a patient frequently leans on their elbow for prolonged periods. The sciatic nerve often becomes entrapped in the pelvis where it emerges from beneath one muscle and crosses over another muscle in the buttock region. This is usually due to prolonged sitting. For the sake of simplicity we will only examine a select few forms of nerve entrapment that affect or mimic back pain.

Entrapment neuropathies are often under recognised and under diagnosed due to their varied and confusing clinical features. Nerves may be injured anywhere along their course throughout the body but they are more prone to compression, entrapment or stretching as they traverse anatomically vulnerable regions, such as near the surface of the skin or in geographically constrained spaces. Early detection and diagnosis of nerve entrapment is essential as the degree and duration of the injury affect the extent of neural recovery and the time taken to heal.

Presentation
Nerve entrapment can result in either radiculopathy (numbness or weakness to the area innervated by the entrapped nerve) or radicular pain

(shooting or lancinating pain that travels down the leg in a band-like pattern), or both. The condition generally only affects the part of the body that is supplied by the nerve that is compressed.

Causes

There are many causes of nerve entrapment. Some examples are tumour (lipoma, neurofibroma, metastasis), pathological conditions (ankylosing spondylitis, aortic aneurysm), disc lesion (herniation, protrusion), myofascial adhesion or compartment syndrome (carpal tunnel syndrome). Certain pathological conditions render nerves more susceptible to entrapment. Diabetes, for example, reduces blood flow to the nerve, which consequently makes the nerve more sensitive to compression.

Diagnosis

Nerve entrapments can be diagnosed using nerve tension tests such as the slump test or straight leg raise (SLR) test. Electrodiagnostic tests include nerve conduction studies and electromyography. Abnormal neurological findings may be associated with decreased muscle strength, impaired sensory system or diminished tendon jerk reflexes. X-rays may show tumour growths, stenosis or infection. CT scan and MRI are necessary to visualise soft-tissue causes of entrapment such as disc protrusion or soft-tissue tumour. There are some entrapments that cannot be seen on any of the current imaging techniques.

Treatment

Nerve entrapments respond well to several forms of myofascial release such as active release techniques and various forms of instrument-assisted myofascial release. These instruments are small, handheld scraping or friction tools. If the entrapment is due to inflammation, drugs such as NSAIDs or steroids that reduce inflammation may be helpful. Surgery may be necessary in some cases that are unresponsive to conservative care. This may involve microdiscectomy for a protruding disc, laminectomy (removal of part of the vertebral lamina) to make space for neural tissue, foraminotomy (enlarging the nerve channel) for the exiting nerve root in the case of foraminal stenosis, or removal of a tumour that was compressing the nerve.

> **Alert**
>
> If a nerve entrapment is left untreated, permanent neurological damage may result.

Sacroiliac joint dysfunction

The sacroiliac (SI) joint is often overlooked as a source of low back pain, but researchers estimate that it accounts for 12 per cent of all chronic low back pain cases. There are various terms used to describe pain stemming from the SI joint: SI joint dysfunction, SI joint syndrome and sacroilitis to name a few. For our purposes we will refer to it as sacroiliac joint dysfunction. Sacroiliac joint pain can be due to either too much (hypermobility) or too little (hypomobility) movement at the joint.

Presentation
Pain tends to occur over one SI joint after straightening up from a stooped position or extending at the lumbar spine. The onset often occurs after a relatively trivial movement such as bending over to pick up something off the floor. The pain may refer down the back of the thigh but rarely past the knee. With an acute strain/sprain of the joint, pain is often sharp or stabbing and is relieved somewhat by sitting or lying. Sources of aggravation often include getting up from a seated position, climbing stairs and rising from a flexed position. During pregnancy up to 80 per cent of women experience some form of SI joint pain.

Causes
Sacroiliac joint dysfunction has various causes such as strain/sprain injury due to the joint being overloaded, such as when a person tries to lift an object that is too heavy. Pregnancy is another cause of sacroiliac dysfunction. During pregnancy the body releases a hormone called relaxin. Relaxin causes muscles and ligaments throughout the body to become looser, which is helpful for the birthing process when the joints of the pelvis need to open up to allow the baby to pass through the birthing canal. However, problems arise if the muscles and ligaments become too slack and instability ensues.

An even worse scenario can occur if the pregnant mother has hypermobility or instability before she became pregnant, with the pregnancy then adding to the situation. Further problems can arise post-delivery if the joints fail to return to their original state (pre-pregnancy) and excessive laxity remains in the joints. The core stability exercises in this book can help overcome the effects of ligament laxity post-pregnancy.

Although the ligaments of the SI joint are some of the strongest in the body, children, pregnant women or those with degenerative diseases are at a greater risk of SI joint dysfunction due to loose SI ligaments. Prolonged flexion or sudden lifting or bending may cause SI joint dysfunction. Twisting injuries or a fall onto the back or buttocks can cause SI joint dysfunction. Other causes include overtraining in athletes, leg length differences, muscular imbalance around the hips or lower back, childhood hip problems, stress fracture of the pelvis, or gait disturbance. Prolonged sitting has also been established as a cause.

Diagnosis

Because sacroiliac joint dysfunction tends to be more of an acute condition, imaging is rarely of any use other than ruling out other causes of low back pain. There are many useful orthopaedic tests that can be performed in clinic by a musculoskeletal practitioner. Although most orthopaedic tests when used alone have relatively low sensitivity and specificity, when several of these tests are positive it provides stronger evidence for the diagnosis. When an appropriate physical examination and history are performed, diagnosis of SI joint dysfunction can be made. The only way to diagnose the condition with 100 per cent certainty is by injecting saline solution into the SI joints, which should reproduce the patient's pain, followed by an injection of a local anaesthetic, which should alleviate the patient's pain.

Treatment

Manual adjusting the SI joint is very effective when the SI joint is subluxated or stuck (hypomobile) and it often results in instant relief of symptoms. Adjustments should be performed cautiously to avoid stretching the SI ligaments on individuals with ligament laxity as further stretching can aggravate the condition. Sacroiliac-belt stabilisation devices are helpful to those with hypermobility or instability. Core-stability muscle exercises have been shown to help stabilise the SI joint in those with joint laxity and resulted in less pain. More recent alternative treatments include platelet-rich plasma injections and prolotherapy, which involves the injection of an irritating solution (like sugar and anaesthetic) into the SI joint space or ligaments to stimulate the healing process. These treatments are still unproven and are not yet universally accepted, so seek a second opinion if you are offered these therapies.

Leg length inequality

Leg-length inequality (LLI) or lower limb–length inequality is quite common. Approximately 10 per cent of the population have up to a 10 mm difference in leg length. It is the most common cause of functional scoliosis and sacroiliac joint problems. The good news is that LLI can be remedied, sometimes quite easily. Some patients only require a heel lift of a few millimetres to correct their LLI, which in turn can correct their spinal scoliosis and may alleviate their low back pain.

Spinal stenosis

The term 'stenosis' comes from the Greek word for choking. In anatomy, stenosis refers to a narrowing of an opening, which can occur in virtually any opening or tube-like structure of the body. In regards to back pain there are two main types of **spinal stenosis**: central canal stenosis and **lateral** foraminal stenosis (also known as lateral recess stenosis).

Patients present with radicular leg pain or neurogenic claudication (pain in the buttocks or legs on walking or standing that resolves with sitting down or bending forward). Symptoms do not occur at rest, but after a patient walks a short distance they begin to experience weakness, tiredness or heaviness in the legs. When walking, a patient generally adopts a stooped forward position and slowly reduces walking speed until they can no longer continue to walk. Radiological evidence of spinal stenosis is also commonly found in the asymptomatic population, thus it is critical that practitioners correlate clinical symptoms and radiological findings before coming up with a definitive diagnosis.

Lateral foraminal stenosis is a narrowing of the opening through which the spinal nerves exit the spinal column. There are two intervertebral foraminae at each spinal level, one on the right side and one on the left. Both central and lateral foraminal stenosis can be due to congenital reasons;

however, symptoms rarely present before a person turns 50, which indicates that it is but one component of the condition. Degenerative lumbar spinal stenosis is the most frequent reason for spinal surgery in patients over 65 years, and 20 per cent of those required reoperation within five years.

Degeneration does not mean pain

Degeneration is a slow and continual process of wear and tear to joints which is not matched by the body's repair processes. Normal degeneration can be hastened by exposure to injury or mechanical stresses. So even relatively young individuals can have advanced degeneration. It has been proven that there is no correlation between radiological signs of joint degeneration in the spine and pain.

Presentation

Patients are generally in their 50s or older, but the condition can present at any age. Patients generally complain of back and lower limb pain. The lower limb pain can occur down a single leg or both legs. Patients complain of the onset of leg cramps while walking that subside after resting for 15 to 20 minutes or by bending over from the waist.

Causes

Spinal stenosis can involve narrowing of the whole spinal canal (central stenosis) or narrowing of the outer part of the canal where the spinal nerves pass (lateral stenosis). The cause can be bony or soft tissue encroachment, and can be either present from birth or acquired. Due to these varied causes, the symptoms can differ greatly. Congenitally, a trefoil (triangular) shape of the spinal canal leads to central canal and lateral stenosis. Acquired stenosis is due to bony outgrowths from the facets, laminae or pedicles, degenerative spondylolisthesis, or enlarged or calcified ligamentum flavum, or both. Postoperative stenosis can result after back surgery (such as laminectomies).

Diagnosis

The symptoms of spinal stenosis can be mimicked by another condition called vascular claudication, which is caused by poor blood flow to the legs. Both conditions cause a cramping leg pain when walking. It is important that a clinician test you to differentiate between the two. This can be done by having you perform a bicycle test. The test involves pedalling on a stationary exercise bicycle while in a forward flexed posture. If your symptoms are due to a lack of blood flow to your legs, you should feel a rapid onset of pain and/or cramping in the legs. If your problem is spinal stenosis, you should feel either no pain at all or a delayed onset of pain long after you commence pedalling. The theory is that in a flexed lumbar position the spinal canal and intervertebral foramina are more open, thus taking pressure off the neurological structures. Patients with clamping due to poor blood flow generally do not have a time delay in the onset of their leg cramps.

X-rays can measure bone-related stenosis; however, CT scans and MRI scans are more useful because they can show soft tissue encroachment.

Treatment

Treatment is based upon the diagnosis of the type and cause of the stenosis. The natural history of the condition seems to suggest that most cases (90 per cent) will have spontaneous resolution of their symptoms without treatment. If attempted, manual manipulation of the spine needs to be done with care, as there is a chance that greater compression of the neural structures can occur—resulting in an exacerbation of symptoms if done inappropriately. The positive response rate for lumbar manipulative therapy was approximately 36 per cent in one study.

Spondylolisthesis

This occurs when there is a bilateral defect in the neural arch of a vertebra, more specifically the pars interarticularis portion, which results in the forward slippage of the involved vertebra on the vertebra below it. There are five forms of spondylolisthesis: isthmic, degenerative, dysplastic, traumatic and pathological. They are grouped based on cause of the pars defect. Spondylolisthesis is graded one to four depending on the degree of vertebral slip—Grade 4 is the greatest degree of displacement. Grade 1 spondylolisthesis generally have few, if any, detectable physical findings. When found, physical changes may include increased lumbar **lordosis** (curvature) or what is termed 'sway back'.

Presentation

For the sake of simplicity we will only address the most common forms of spondylolisthesis—namely, **isthmic** in the younger population and **degenerative** in the older population.

Isthmic: for Grade 1 spondylolisthesis, patients may be asymptomatic or have generalised low back pain made worse by lumbar extension. Grade 2–4 spondylolisthesis have more obvious physical findings such as an accentuated lumbar lordosis (which may extend up into the lower thoracic spine). A highly diagnostic abnormal gait pattern, called the pelvic waddle, may be present. It is characterised by a stiff legged short stride gait associated with pelvic rotation on each step. It is uncommon to come across any lower limb neurological findings such as pins and needles, numbness or muscle weakness.

Degenerative: this may be asymptomatic or may cause signs and symptoms of spinal-canal narrowing (stenosis), which include back and lower limb pain. The lower limb pain can occur down a single leg or both legs. Patients complain of the onset of leg cramps while walking that subside after resting for 15 to 20 minutes or by bending forward from the waist.

Diagnosis

The most common method of diagnosis is X-ray, and lateral views will often display the forward slippage. Oblique X-ray views of both the right and left sides are the best ways to visualise the actual break (pars defects). Stability of a spondylolisthesis may be assessed by a traction (patient hangs from a bar) or compression radiograph (a 20-kilogram backpack on the shoulders). Physical examination may reveal a 'step defect', which may be visualised or palpated in the lumbar spine, but is not always present in all cases. Some orthopaedic tests such as the single-leg standing hyperextension test (stork test) are useful, and this test is considered positive if it reproduces the patient's low back pain.

Grading of spondylolisthesis is done by using lateral view radiographs by dividing the sacrum or **inferior** vertebra into quarters. Each quarter represents a grade, thus a slippage of 0 to 25 per cent is a Grade 1, slippage of 26 to 50 per cent is a Grade 2, slippage of 51 to 75 per cent is a Grade 3 and slippage of more than 75 per cent is a Grade 4. Some researchers also recognise a Grade 5, which is when the slippage is greater than 100 per cent. A SPECT bone scan can be done to identify a spondylolisthesis that is not yet visible on an X-ray.

Causes

The isthmic spondylolisthesis is caused by biomechanical stress; it is believed that the repetitive forces imparted on the pars interarticularis results in fatigue fracture. There is a correlation between spondylolisthesis and sports that emphasis repetitive lumbar hyperextension such as gymnastics and bowling in cricket.

Treatment

Most Grade 1 spondylolistheses are stable and not symptomatic, and thus do not require special treatment. Conservative treatment involves restriction of physical activity, strengthening exercises for abdominal and back muscles, bedrest, low-back bracing and non-narcotic analgesics. Research indicates favourable response to manual manipulation, when either the sacroiliac joint or the lumbar facet joints above the involved segment are manipulated. Many spondylolisthesis patients have concurrent facet joint syndrome, hyperlordosis or sacral fixation, or both. It is often these conditions that are the actual source of their symptoms, not the spondylolisthesis itself. Therefore, treatment of these secondary conditions often helps resolve symptoms of low back pain.

For patients found to have a hot spot on their bone scan, a back brace that limits backward-bending can be worn for several weeks to prevent a pars defect from occurring. The Boston overlap brace is an example of such a brace. It immobilises the spine while allowing full activities including sports. When used in conjunction with flexibility and muscle-strengthening exercises it can successfully manage pain in over 80 per cent of patients under the age of 30.

Recommendations

If a spondylolisthesis is present or suspected, avoid activities that require repetitive lumbar hyperextension. If the condition is new, get compression

---

Alert

Any activity involving repeated hyperextension of the spine is likely to aggravate spondylolisthetic symptoms. This includes sport, work and exercises.

---

and distraction X-rays taken in order to ascertain whether the spondylolis-thesis is stable or unstable. An unstable case may require surgery to prevent nerve damage.

Vertebral endplate fracture

When the spinal column is compressed vertically, the walls of the vertebrae remain rigid and the nucleus of the disc pressurises and cause the endplates of the vertebrae to bulge inward, which then compresses the inner spongy bone of the vertebral body. Vertebral endplates are the first component of the spine to fail due to compression.

Endplate fractures are a common cause of low back pain, but they are seldom diagnosed by practitioners. In the elderly, the vertebral endplate often detaches from its underlying bone; this is thought to be due a loss of internal pressure that compresses the endplate against the vertebral body.

A functionally important structural linkage is formed between the disc and adjacent vertebrae via the vertebral endplate. Endplates separate the vertebral bone from the disc itself and prevent the highly hydrated nucleus from bulging into the adjacent vertebrae.

Upon reaching skeletal maturity, the cartilage of the endplate under-goes substantial remodelling and reabsorption that results in the cartilage being replaced by bone. Of note is the fact that this remodelling results in decreased diffusion and nutrient exchange between vertebral body bone marrow and the disc, thus the disc receives less nutrients in the adult spine.

Research indicates that the weakest point of the vertebral endplate is where disc fibres insert into the vertebral body at the outer edge of the endplate. It is the most common site for fracture in adolescents.

Presentation
Vertebral endplate fracture (VEF) may be asymptomatic. In symptomatic cases there is often localised, non-radiating low back pain and local ten-derness of sudden onset.

Causes
The most common cause of VEF is traumatic spinal loading. The forces required to cause VEF can occur with a sudden fall, landing on the

buttocks or forceful muscle activity. Predisposition for VEF include cancers such as multiple myeloma and metastasis, disc space infections, discitis or other processes that can weaken the endplate or the underlying bone. Another cause of VEF are fatigue fractures due to repetitive spinal compression or compression with flexion. It has been shown that endplates can fracture when loaded to between 50 per cent and 80 per cent of their maximal strength with as few as 100 repetitions. For example, a factory worker bending over to lift a 20-kilogram object one hundred times per day could end up with an endplate fracture. Loads of this magnitude are commonly encountered in normal working demands.

Diagnosis
Vertebral endplate fracture can sometimes be seen on lateral X-rays. CT scans and MRI scans consistently demonstrate endplate fractures.

Treatment
Generally endplate fractures heal on their own without treatment or intervention. Physical exercise and training can strengthen the vertebral bodies, making them better able to withstand larger vertical loads. It should be noted that careful exercise planning is necessary, as there are risks of endplate fracture if the patient attempts to take on a lifting task that exceeds their vertebral endplate capacity.

Complications
VEF can lead to internal disc derangement (see section on internal disc derangement).

Recommendations
Avoid repetitive bending while lifting or carrying heavy items. An example of this is shovelling a heavy material in a flexed position for a long period of time.

Alert

Any exercises that heavily load the spine may prolong recovery or cause further injury.

Vertebral compression fracture

When discussing a vertebral compression fracture of the spine, the vertebral body is the component of the vertebra that is fractured and becomes compressed. Compression fractures tend to occur in individuals with decreased bone density. They may occur in individuals with normal bone density; however, the cases are rare and often require large forces. Osteopenia and osteoporosis are both forms of decreased bone density. While the cause of osteopenia or osteoporosis can be various pathological diseases, often the actual cause of the decreased bone density is not identified and the patient is simply given a calcium supplement to treat the symptom of decreased bone density. The problem with this approach is that if the cause of the decreased bone density is not identified, the patient will take calcium supplements forever in order to maintain their bone density. A secondary problem is that although calcium supplements increase one's bone density, they can actually make bones more brittle and sometimes more susceptible to fractures.

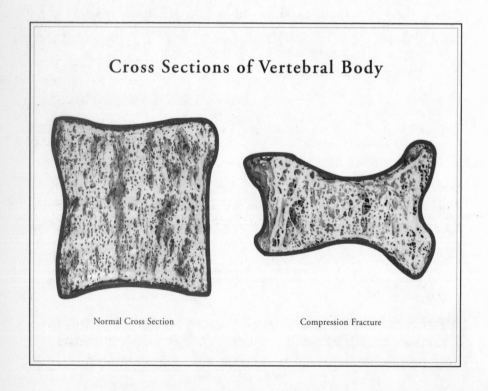

Cross Sections of Vertebral Body

Normal Cross Section   Compression Fracture

Alert

Any manual therapy on a fractured vertebra is not recommended. Open surgery can be risky for older patients because of poor bone repair as well as the presence of other conditions. Steroid drug therapies are associated with long-term bone loss.

The actual source of pain from vertebra compression fractures is not fully understood. Theories suggest that either the fascia surrounding the vertebral body or the blood vessels within the vertebral body cause the pain. Either way the pain of the compression fracture is temporary, usually lasting four to twelve weeks; however, the structural change to the vertebral body is permanent.

Approximately two-thirds of VCFs go undiagnosed because older individuals often think that back pain is merely part of ageing or due to arthritis.

Many people are unaware that it is actually bone quality, not bone quantity, that is the most important variable for preventing compression fractures. Vertebral bodies are the primary shock absorbers of the spine, contrary to what most textbooks teach about spine mechanics and physiology. Thus, once vertebral bodies undergo a compression fracture, their shape is permanently altered and the entire spine becomes less tolerant of loads. With age we tend to lose bony struts, called trabeculae, within our vertebral bodies.

There is currently much confusion regarding calcium supplementation for the prevention of osteoporotic fractures, which is reflected by the wide range of daily intake recommendations made around the world: 700 mg in the United Kingdom, 800 mg in Scandinavia, 1200 mg in the United States and 1300 mg in Australia and New Zealand. Recent studies have even shown that high-dose calcium supplementation can have negative effects such as increased risk of stroke and cardiovascular events. Other studies have shown increased risk of bone fracture with high-calcium supplementation.

Osteoporosis or osteopenia?

Most people are familiar with the term osteoporosis, which means bones becoming porous. It is a bone disorder characterised by abnormal loss of bone density and deterioration of bone tissue, with an increased fracture risk. It occurs most often in post-menopausal women, sedentary or immobilised individuals and patients on long-term steroid therapy.

There is a lesser known precursor to osteoporosis called osteopenia. The word osteopenia means 'poverty of bone'. Osteopenia is a condition of sub-normally mineralised bone, usually the result of a rate of bone breakdown that exceeds the rate of bone formation.

Osteopenia can also be a sign in other diseases that diminish bone mass, such as osteomalacia, hyperparathyroidism and rickets.

Both osteopenia and osteoporosis can be diagnosed by X-ray, CT scan, MRI scans and various bone-density scans. The diagnosis of either condition does not tell us the cause of the decreased bone density. Further testing must be carried out to figure out the cause.

Did you know that:

- One in three women will develop osteoporosis
- One in twelve men will develop osteoporosis
- After the age of 80, the number of men affected equals the number of women?

Presentation

Vertebral compression fractures may or may not be symptomatic. For those without symptoms, the patient often is unaware they had the fracture until they undergo spinal imaging. Symptomatic patients often suffer immediate moderate to severe localised back pain after a specific incident. Patients are usually 50 years of age or older, and more commonly women (particularly postmenopausal women). Decreased physical height occurs because compression fractures decrease the length of the spine. Multiple compression fractures lead to a hyperkyphotic (rounded) spine or dowager's hump. Those with a small or thin frame have an increased risk of osteoporosis and thus VCF.

Causes

The most common cause of VCF is osteoporosis, which may be due to various diseases (see section on osteoporosis). When osteoporosis is present, bones become brittle, so even fairly low-force events may cause a fracture. These include activities such as lifting an object, stepping off a curb, missing a step or even coughing and sneezing. Sometimes it takes many of these events, which cause multiple microscopic breaks in the internal bony architecture of the vertebral body, to occur before the entire vertebral body collapses, which results in a compression fracture. As more VCFs occur, the more hunched over the patient becomes, which can contribute to subsequent fractures.

Other causes include poor nutrition or poor digestion, trauma, long-term corticosteroid use and bone-weakening diseases such as bone cancer.

Diagnosis

Lateral X-rays of the spine are the easiest and most cost-effective way of evaluating the spine for compression fractures. A compression fracture is diagnosed if there is greater than 15 per cent decrease in the vertebral body height. If a compression fracture is present, often the patient is referred for a bone density test to rule out osteoporosis. The patient may have focal tenderness to touch at the level of the VCF. Early diagnosis is important because if the cause of the VFC is identified, future fractures of this type possibly can be prevented. Sometimes VCF is the first indication of cancer, thus it is extremely important to ascertain the cause of the VFC. Often further investigation is required, including pathology testing.

Treatment

Conservative care such as anti-inflammatories, analgesics, opiods, ice-packs or heat-packs (depending on which one gives better pain relief) rest, bracing and physical therapy are indicated for those without neurological impairment. If you don't respond to conservative care, medical procedures are available that can help. Currently the most commonly performed medical procedures are kyphoplasty and percutaneous vertebroplasty (PV). Kyphoplasty involves inserting a tiny balloon into the vertebral body to expand it, with the space then filled with bone cement and the balloon withdrawn. PV involves injecting bone cement into the vertebral compression fracture without the use of a balloon. The PV stabilises the fractured vertebral body and provides immediate reduction or relief of pain caused by the fracture. Although this process involves a major surgical procedure, the level of technology and surgeon skill makes these operations usually very successful. Risks of kyphoplasty and PV include the possibility of mechanical compression of the spinal cord with cement leakage, tissue damage, blood clots in the lung, and respiratory failure. Surgery may be required if you have progressive neurological impairment or spinal instability.

If your VCF is due to osteoporosis, tests to determine any nutrient (vitamins and minerals) deficiencies need to be performed. Once a deficiency is identified, conditions which can cause a deficiency need to be ruled out. If the deficiency is simply due to poor nutrition, appropriate dietary changes can be made. If deficiencies cannot be fixed through dietary changes, supplements can be used.

Recommendations

If the VCF is due to osteoporosis, finding out the cause of the osteoporosis is paramount. If the cause is a calcium deficiency, that does not simply mean taking more calcium. For some people the cause of their calcium deficiency may be due to deficiency in vitamin D, which absorbs calcium from the intestine. For others, the cause may be irritable bowel syndrome, which can cause poor calcium absorption. Both these problems involve calcium; however, neither will respond to a calcium supplement because the calcium will still fail to get absorbed from the intestine. The correct approach for the first example would be to increase vitamin D intake via diet, supplementation or sun exposure. In the second example, the cause of the irritable bowel syndrome needs to be identified and treated before calcium will begin to be absorbed effectively. Exercise, specifically resistance training, has been repeatedly shown to be effective in increasing bone density. However, a well-designed exercise program is necessary in order to safely and effectively increase bone density. If the patient has osteoporosis and is being treated by physical therapy such as spinal manipulation, only low-force techniques should be used. Avoid using heat over the fractured area within the first few days after the injury, as it may cause excessive inflammation.

Vitamin D

Vitamin D plays an important health role, but we still don't fully understand all of its functions within the body. We do know it helps absorption of calcium from the digestive tract to be used in bones and other tissues. Sun exposure stimulates the skin to create vitamin D. Optimal levels of circulating vitamin D range from 30 to 90 ng/mL. We require between 3 and 20 minutes of sun exposure each day, depending on the season and our skin type. Vitamin D deficiency has been shown to increase the risk of osteoporotic fractures. Low levels of vitamin D is associated with malabsorption of calcium, which results in bone density loss. The daily recommended supplemental dose of vitamin D is around 200IU to 400IU but higher doses have been recommended in order to prevent osteoporotic fractures.

Coccydynia

Coccydynia is defined as pain in or around the coccyx (tailbone) without any significant radiation or associated low back pain, with triggering or worsening of the pain when sitting (or, more rarely, on moving from the sitting to the standing position). Coccydynia is not a very common cause of low back pain; it is actually a symptom, not a diagnosis.

Coccydynia is more common in women because the coccyx is more exposed than in men, women have a wider pelvis (which places more pressure on the coccyx) than men, and because the injury commonly occurs during childbirth. During delivery, the baby's head passes over the top of the coccyx, and the pressure created between the coccyx and the baby's head can sometimes damage the tailbone structures (the disc, ligaments and bones).

A coccygeal spicule, an abnormal bony outgrowth found on the back of the coccyx, has been identified as a source of coccydynia. Because the spicule protrudes backwards, it reduces the surface area of the coccyx that normally comes into contact when a person is sitting. This significantly increases the force being placed on a small area when sitting, resulting in pain. It is more commonly found in immobile parts of the coccyx, in which the pressure from the spicule is made worse by the coccyx being unable to move out of the way. Spicules are not injury-related, which explains many non-traumatic causes of coccydynia. Sufferers who are carrying less body weight can feel pain due to less subcutaneous fat cushioning the coccyx.

Presentation

Coccydynia presents as localised pain at the very bottom of the spine in the region just above the anus. Patients may also get shooting referral pain into the posterior thighs, pain during bowel movements or pain during sex. Pain is usually made worse by sitting or any activity that increases pressure on the coccyx. It is far more common in women than men. Pain may be made worse with constipation and can lessen after a bowel movement. Pain can be aggravated when moving from a sitting to standing position.

Treatment

Generally coccydynia is a self-limiting condition that will get better over the course of several weeks without treatment. However, for those cases that do not self-resolve, there are several available treatments, depending on the cause. Mechanical causes of coccydynia have been shown to respond well to spinal manipulation/mobilisation as well as soft tissue therapy. Treatments that reduce pain (acupuncture, cold pack, analgesics, NSAIDs) and activity modification that reduces the pressure being placed on the coccyx are often sufficient to alleviate pain. Use of a 'donut pillow' or a U-shaped pillow can be helpful because it takes pressure off the coccyx while sitting. If pain is caused or increased with bowel movements or constipation, stool softeners and increased fibre and water intake can be helpful. A local injection of anaesthetic or corticosteroid has been shown to alleviate patients' symptoms from one week to several years. In extremely rare cases, surgery to remove part of the coccyx or the entire coccyx (coccygectomy) may be recommended. However, this is only considered if the pain has been unresponsive to conservative therapy and the patient's pain is severe and has lasted for at least several months without change.

Causes

Local trauma such as falling onto the coccyx, giving birth, or prolonged sitting on a hard surface (such as horseback riding) can cause this condition. Trauma to the coccyx can cause strain or tearing of surrounding muscles or sprain of local ligaments, both of which can produce pain. Coccygeal instability due to trauma can cause the coccyx to luxate (abnormally shift) forward or backward, producing pain in the coccyx area. The formation of a coccygeal spicule can be a cause of coccydynia. More rare causes include bone infection (osteomyelitis) or a tumour of the coccyx. Coccydynia can also be idiopathic, meaning the cause is unknown.

Diagnosis

In some cases, where previous diagnostic images are available, they may be compared to current images to measure any structural changes over time. One study demonstrated that dynamic lateral radiographs (comparing coccyx position during sitting compared to standing) was capable of discerning a cause of coccydynia in 69 per cent of a sample group. Currently the gold standard for diagnosing coccydynia is anaesthetic blocks, with an injection administered near the coccyx. If positive, the patient's pain should be temporarily eliminated or at least significantly reduced.

Physical examination includes feeling the coccyx and its surrounding structures, if the coccyx is not too tender. When a spicule (bony growth) is present, it can easily be felt through the skin. Most patients presenting with a spicule show evidence of an infection adjacent to the coccyx. There is a chance that a pelvic or a rectal exam needs to take place to check for a mass or tumour.

Complications

Surgery (coccygectomy) only has an 80–90 per cent success rate, and there is a long and painful healing process that can vary from three months to a year. There is also the risk of local infection or damaging the rectum, which sits directly in front of the coccyx.

Multiple causes of back pain

Some good news regarding back pain is that having multiple sources of pain in one patient is uncommon. Studies on low back pain indicate that patients tend to have a single condition in isolation as the cause of their back pain. Fewer than 5 per cent of chronic low back pain patients have more than one source of back pain.

My back pain story
Rener Gracie

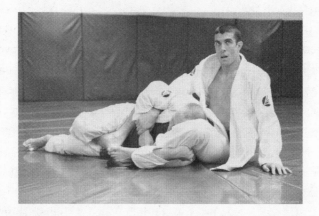

You would have never guessed that a young and fit 19-year-old man would suffer from debilitating low back pain, particularly if that individual was one of the top Brazilian Jiu-Jitsu martial artists in the world. However, for Rener Gracie, this was a reality.

Having come from a family of sporting legends, Rener Gracie was introduced to the sport Brazilian Jiu-Jitsu (BJJ) at a very young age. While his BJJ training imparted him with abilities such as improved body awareness, balance, flexibility and strength, the down side was that he would often place his spine in precarious positions. At 19 years of age, Rener began experiencing bouts of searing pain in his right thigh and buttock. Being young, he hoped that the pain would just go away on its own, but this did not happen. For months he endured chronic daily pain in his right leg, which continued to progress in severity—restricting his ability to train and compete in his sport. Eventually the pain became unbearable, and Rener was barely able to walk due to pain. He consulted one of the best spinal surgeons in California and, after an MRI of his lumbar spine, the cause of Rener's excruciating leg pain was discovered. It was a 6 mm disc herniation causing irritation of a spinal nerve. The surgeon recommended Rener be scheduled for immediate back surgery. A week later, Rener underwent back surgery to remove the herniation.

Although the surgery was successful, Rener could still feel some mild remnant pain in the same part of his thigh as before. Soon after surgery Rener undertook a vigorous regimen of back rehabilitation with a physiotherapist, which consisted of four to five treatments per week. The physio taught Rener about the importance of a stable spine and introduced him to core stability exercises that would restore and rebuild his low back. Six months later, Rener felt that his back was strong again; however, he was fearful of re-injuring his low back while training, so he took an additional four months to further rehabilitate his low back. Nearly one year after having back surgery, Rener's back was stronger than it had ever been and he began training, teaching and competing in BJJ again. He continued to maintain a daily routine of core stability exercises, to which he attributes the success of his recovery. Ten years post–back surgery, Rener continues to train and teach the sport he loves at the Gracie Academy in Torrance, California. He remains free of back pain by maintaining a routine of monthly treatments at a spinal care clinic that specialises in conservative spinal care, and his daily routine of core stability exercises.

Rener Gracie is a head instructor at the Gracie Jiu-Jitsu Academy and cocreator of the Gracie University, the world's largest online Jiu-Jitsu training program. He is the grandson of Helio Gracie, the creator of Brazilian Jiu-Jitsu, and the son of Rorion Gracie, who co-founded the hugely popular Ultimate Fighting Championship (UFC).

3 Diagnosis of back pain: history-taking, testing and diagnostic imaging

History-taking

When a patient presents to a healthcare professional for the treatment of a back problem, the first steps which must be taken involve a diagnostic assessment. This starts with a history-taking and is followed by a physical assessment. Contrary to popular view, the history-taking interview is often the most important part of a diagnostic assessment. It is essential that it be thorough enough to be able to categorise the nature of the problem, identify the organs or body tissues involved and then hopefully identify the specific source of the problem. History-taking should not involve the filling out of a questionnaire or the posing of a pre-determined list of standardised questions. The best history is obtained using a dynamic process where each new question is based on the answer to the question that precedes it. History-taking is a detective process of problem-solving where clinicians combine their knowledge of anatomy and normal function with an understanding of the disease process, and use their experience to solve the cause of the back problem.

Typically, history-taking in patients with low back pain has the initial goal of establishing whether the back pain is due to either a red flag condition (pathology), a nerve-root compression problem (**radiculopathy**) or a mechanical cause. This is because these three broad categories of problems have very different management paths. In Chapter 2 we outlined the types of symptoms that could indicate red-flag conditions. Remember, such conditions require medical or hospital assessment without delay as they may be related to serious or life-threatening conditions. It should be noted that red-flag conditions cause less than 2 per cent of back pain cases.

Once the likelihood of a red-flag condition has been eliminated, the role of the history is to categorise the nature of the problem. Broadly speaking, most back pain is related to either trauma, degeneration, developmental disorders, infection or tumour. As infections and tumours are red-flag conditions, their possibility should have been eliminated early on in the history-taking. After the most likely category of the problem is identified, questions are asked to uncover the location of the problem and the most probable cause. The specific tissues involved in the problem may not be identified from the history. That is covered by the physical examination and is outlined below. Additionally, the history-taking is used to identify 'yellow flags'. Yellow flags are situations which impact adversely on the ability of a patient to get well quickly. They usually involve psychosocial problems such as work or family stress, impending legal action, the presence of co-existing health problems (such as diabetes), and adverse habits such as smoking, drinking or use of other recreational drugs.

Good clinicians take a history that is detailed and searching, but always focused on solving the problem of the cause of the back pain and its most likely solution. Always be sceptical of a therapist who takes little time or pays little attention to your clinical history.

Physical examination

Physical examination is an important part of the diagnostic process. Just like history-taking, it should not be a standardised or prefabricated set of manoeuvres applied to all patients but should be tailor-made for the patient at hand. The correct tests to perform are determined after careful consideration of the history-taking findings. A good history leads to clear suspicions of the disease process and body tissues most likely involved. The physical examination entails testing of suspect tissues for normal function and tenderness. It is usually the case that the better the history, the fewer tests needed in the physical examination. For example, if history-taking suggests that a ligament injury is present, the physical examination centres on stress-testing the ligaments in the low back. As well as this, a good diagnostician will also confirm that structures other than ligaments are not involved by testing neighbouring tissues.

The use of specific tests in the physical examination of low back pain patients has caused some controversy. This is for two reasons. Firstly there is the mistaken belief that it is usually impossible to differentiate between the different causes of mechanical back pain. Secondly, the tests themselves are not fully reliable when used individually. The best clinicians do use physical examination tests, and rely on the findings of *several* such tests—never on any one test. In this way, by looking for corroboration between various test findings, good clinicians can make diagnoses with reasonable confidence.

Another important use for physical examination is to ensure and measure progress. During physical-examination testing, commonly the clinician will find a test that gives a strong 'positive' result. Usually this means that the test elicits a painful reaction when applied. Clinicians record this finding and periodically reapply the test to see if it still elicits the same finding over time or after treatment. Typically a patient with a very painful positive-test finding will progressively experience less pain over time as they get better. Ideally treatment strategies can change and milestones can be set to coincide with such changes. For instance, a patient who has back pain with leg pain may be placed on an intensive treatment program initially. Imagine that the patient has sharp leg pain on raising their leg while lying down. A clinician may decide that intensive treatment should continue until the patient can raise the leg without reproducing pain. In this way the test (raising the leg and reproducing pain) is used to set a milestone which, once achieved, will change the intensity of treatment. Used this way, such tests are called 'tag tests'. If a patient has a tag-test finding that is not improving, or is getting worse, this is a strong indicator that the current treatment strategy needs to be carefully reassessed.

Look for a therapist who uses physical examination in a purposeful way to find structures or movements that are not functioning or are painful. Good clinicians use some testing at each and every visit to ensure and monitor progress. Avoid therapists who don't appear to use physical testing in these ways.

Radiologists

These are medical doctors who specialise in radiographic imaging, which includes X-rays, CT scans, nuclear medicine, MRI scan or PET scan to diagnose or treat medical conditions. Some radiologists do further training to be able to perform interventional radiology (injections guided with the use of radiologic imaging), which can be used for purposes of treatment or diagnosis. Since radiologists specialise in imaging they can be very helpful to practitioners when working on diagnosing a patient. A radiologist can recommend to a practitioner which imaging modality is most appropriate for the patient, based on clinical findings and differential diagnosis.

It is often a radiographer (radiology technologist) who positions the patient and takes the image. However, it is the radiologist who examines the images and produces a report of their findings which is then sent to the referring practitioner along with a copy of the images.

Radiography

This is a technology that uses X-rays to view the internal structures of the body. An X-ray generator produces X-rays, which are then passed through a person; some of the X-rays will be absorbed by the body. Those that pass through are recognised by a detector or sensitised film behind the patient. It then forms an image called a radiograph, or more commonly an 'X-ray'. X-rays are a form of electromagnetic radiation. They were discovered by Wilhelm Roentgen in 1895, and he chose an 'X' to signify an unknown type of radiation. He discovered them by accident while experimenting with electron beams in a gas discharge tube. While working with the beam Roentgen noticed that a plate across the room covered with barium plati-nocyanoide began to fluoresce (glow). This fascinated Roentgen because the discharge tube was surrounded by heavy black cardboard, which he assumed would block the most of the radiation. Roentgen then began feverishly experimenting with X-rays, defining their properties and characteristics. Professor Roentgen produced the first radiograph, an image of his wife's hand, on 8 November 1895. In recognition for his discovery, Roentgen was awarded the first Nobel Prize for Physics in 1901.

Historically, X-ray images have required film, various chemicals used in the development of the film and a darkroom to develop the images. Nowadays, most radiology clinics have switched to digital X-ray machines, which do not require developing, eliminating the need for a darkroom and so saving massive amounts of time. Another benefit of digital X-rays is that they can be viewed immediately. This allows the radiologist the opportunity to retake the picture if the image is not clear. Before digital X-rays the radiologist would have had to develop the film at a later time, which meant that if it was a poor-quality image, the patient would be required to come back for another X-ray.

Standard X-rays do not show soft tissue clearly so a contrast medium can be introduced to outline certain structures. Contrast media are liquids that absorb more X-rays than the surrounding tissue. Contrast media can be ingested to outline organs over the digestive tract or injected into the bloodstream to examine blood vessels. X-rays have been made much safer than in the past by reducing the patient's exposure to radiation. In the 1940s X-ray dosages often were 50 to 100 times higher than those used today. A referral from your practitioner is required in order to have an X-ray taken. Those practitioners who can refer for an X-ray in Australia are chiropractors, osteopaths, dentists, general practitioners, medical doctors, physiotherapists and podiatrists (only lower limb).

X-ray

Reasons to have this test
Bone fracture, dislocation, metastasis, neoplasm and infection. Joint degeneration, arthrosis and spatial alignment problems.

Reasons you might not be able to have this test
X-rays use ionising radiation, which has been linked to an increased risk of cancer. For most plain X-rays, the radiation dose is no more than the ionising radiation from normal environmental background over a period of four days. There are no absolute dangers. Pregnancy is a **relative contraindication** due to the risk to the developing embryo. Side effects include birth defects and cancer.

Positive attributes
X-rays are often the first line of choice for imaging due to their speed, wide availability and low cost. X-rays are relatively inexpensive compared to other imaging techniques such a CT scans and MRI scans. Standard X-rays have relatively low radiation amounts compared to CT scans. The process of taking X-rays is much faster than CT scans and MRI scans.

Negative attributes

X-rays use ionising radiation. X-rays do not show soft-tissue structures and, therefore, are not useful for the diagnosis of most soft-tissue related conditions. Despite what many believe, discs, which are soft tissue, cannot be visualised or diagnosed on a standard X-ray. X-rays should not be taken of pregnant women, so other imaging methods which can be more expensive or time consuming may be necessary. Practitioners may be unaware that a patient has previously had a particular area imaged in the past and may order a repeat X-ray of the same area. This unnecessarily exposes the patient to more radiation without providing any further clinical information. It can be difficult to properly X-ray extremely large or obese individuals because fewer X-rays pass through the patient, resulting in poor-image quality.

Recommendations

Remove all metallic objects or piercings prior to being X-rayed. Be as still as possible while being X-rayed, as movement can blur the image and force the radiographer to repeat the image, which exposes you to more radiation. Be sure to advise the radiographer if you have had previous imaging of the same area, as this can avoid the same area being imaged unnecessarily. Females must advise the radiographer if they are pregnant or think they could be.

X-ray only when clinically indicated

There has to be a medical reason to X-ray someone. There are industry guidelines that practitioners are meant to follow when referring for X-rays. Next time you see a new practitioner and they want to X-ray you straightaway, ask them why you need one. If they can't give you a straight answer, it is likely that they don't have a clinically viable **indication** for requesting an X-ray, and you may not need to be X-rayed.

Computer tomography (CT)

A computer tomography (CT) scan uses multiple X-rays to rapidly take multiple images and compile them into complete cross-sectional 'slices' of soft tissue, bone and blood vessels. CT scans can visualise areas of the body that cannot be seen with standard X-ray imaging. Therefore, CT scans often result in earlier diagnosis and more successful treatment of many diseases such as brain injuries and cancer.

A CT scanner consists of an X-ray source, radiation detectors and electronic devices mounted on a frame or gantry that surrounds the patient.

Reasons to have this test
Trauma, infection, neoplasms, vascular conditions, congenital conditions, arthritic conditions and intervertebral disc conditions, soft-tissue lesions and numerous diseases are possible indications.

Reasons you might not be able to have this test
There are few **contraindications** for the use of CT scans. As with other imaging techniques that employ ionising radiation, patient dose must be kept as low as possible. The risk of exposure to any type of medical ionising radiation needs to be weighed against the potential gain from the information obtained from the imaging. Hypersensitivity to iodine products, delayed renal clearance and congestive heart failure contraindicate the use of some contrast-infusion techniques. If intravenous contrast is to be used, patients with diabetes, renal compromise and congestive heart failure should be cautiously evaluated. Blood urea/nitrogen and creatinine laboratory tests should be performed on every patient prior to using intravenous contrast. If these tests are abnormal, contrast infusion is contraindicated.

Positive attributes
CT scans provide much higher detail of bone outline and structure compared to plain X-ray. CT scanners are less claustrophobic than MRI scanners because the scanning unit is not fully enclosed.

Negative attributes
CT scanning uses ionising radiation at doses that can be 100 times greater than plain X-rays. In order to produce the best image, higher radiation exposure is necessary. CT scans should not be taken of pregnant women. CT scanning is useful in the lumbar spine but the lack of epidural fat in the cervical and thoracic spine prohibits adequate CT visualisation of disc herniations in those regions unless contrast is used.

Recommendations

Remove all metallic objects prior to scan as they will cause poor imaging due to beam scattering. Those who suffer from a high level of claustrophobia may not be able to be scanned. Children should not be scanned without strong clinical indications. There are two major concerns regarding exposing children to ionising radiation. The first is that they are growing rapidly, providing a greater opportunity for radiation to disrupt cell development. The second concern is that children have a longer life expectancy, giving a longer time for any radiation damage effects, if present, to influence long-term health.

Magnetic resonance imaging (MRI)

An MRI scan is a relatively new diagnostic tool used in radiology to visualise internal structures of the body. MRI machines use a combination of magnetic fields and radio waves to look at hydrogen-atom vibrations in the body. The magnetic field causes the hydrogen atoms to align like the needle of a compass; radio waves are then introduced into the body, which are absorbed by the hydrogen proton. Energy is released after 'exciting' the hydrogen molecules, which is recognised by a coil in the machine. These energy signals are then calculated using a high-powered computer to produce three-dimensional images of the body.

Reasons to have this test

MRI can be useful in cases of trauma, infection, tumours, vascular conditions, congenital conditions, arthritic conditions, intervertebral disc lesions, soft tissue lesion and numerous diseases.

Reasons you might not be able to have this test

Patients with claustrophobia, pacemakers, aneurysm clips, metallic splinters in the eye and dental implants (if magnetic) cannot be scanned. There is a risk that pacemakers may malfunction during the scan. Aneurysm clips in the brain can dislodge, which then tears the artery that they were placed on to repair. Most modern surgical implants such as artificial joints, surgical clips and heart stents are made of non-magnetic materials, which can be safely scanned. Even some magnetic materials may be approved for scanning by a radiologist.

Negative attributes

The machine has a fairly small diameter tube (60 cm) for patients to occupy; very large individuals who may not fit into the machine cannot be scanned. It can be claustrophobic for certain individuals and is very noisy. Medical sedatives can be provided in some settings. The patient must remain very still during the entire procedure, which can take 20 to 90 minutes or more, depending on the area being examined. If the patient moves even slightly, the process may have to be repeated. The cost of the exam is relatively high compared to other diagnostic imaging procedures. This is due to the fact that the machines are expensive to purchase (each costing a few million dollars) and maintain. Most clinics opt not to image pregnant women if possible, as there is little research into the effects of strong magnetic fields on the developing foetus.

Positive attributes

MRI is safe, non-invasive and does not cause pain. It is currently the gold standard for soft-tissue imaging. Unlike X-rays or CT scans, MRI has no ionising radiation and there are no known biological hazards to humans from being exposed to magnetic fields of the strength used by MRI technology. It can image in any plane, whereas CT is limited to one plane, the axial plane. Once you're out of the machine your body and its chemistry return to normal. New 'open MR imager' machines allow many claustrophobic patients to be examined. Unlike X-rays, there is no concern about the image quality being adversely affected by the size of the patient. MRI provides superior spatial and contrast resolution and is the best imaging modality for evaluating bone marrow and contents of the spinal canal. MRI also has the advantage of being able to identify areas of active inflammation, which appear as brighter areas on the images. This allows radiologists to differentiate between older, resolved problems and active, new ones.

Recommendations

Claustrophobic patients can request a sedative be administered prior to the scan (normally only done in hospital settings), or some radiology clinics now have MRI scanners that are open at the sides. MRI is often the diagnostic follow-up if X-ray or CT scanning or both fail to provide sufficient information.

Myelography

Myelography is defined as radiographic visualisation of the spinal cord after injection of a contrast dye into the spinal subarachnoid space just next to the cord. The contrast medium used is water-soluble. Currently CT myelography (CTM) is used more often than plain film myelography as it provides greater image detail. For a lumbar spine myelography examination the patient must first have the injection followed by a four- to six-hour waiting period. Then the patient is brought back for the X-ray or CT scan. Before the evolution of CT and MRI, myelograms were the only method of imaging the spinal cord and central canal contents.

Reasons to have this test
Myelograms are used to detect many spinal-column pathologies, including arthritis, tuberculosis, herniated disc, nerve-root injury, secondary or metastatic tumours, some primary spinal tumours and spinal cord cysts.

Reasons you might not be able to have this test
Patients on tricyclic antidepressants, monoamine oxidase inhibitors and phenothiazine medications. Patients with a history of seizures require prophylactic medication before examination. Those with an allergy to iodine or signs of dehydration should not be given a myelogram. All patients should be tested for iodine sensitivity before the procedure.

Positive attributes
The main benefit of myelography is that it outlines the margins of the spinal canal contents. CTM is useful for evaluating nerve-root sheaths, the cauda equina, pathology of surrounding bone and joints, and shape and size of the spinal canal, and it can be used to review post-operative changes. Since it can be a dynamic test, myelography is excellent for assessing the stability of the spine, particularly with spondylolisthesis.

Negative attributes

A high dose of ionising radiation is used. Long waiting period between the time of injection and imaging time are inconvenient and delays diagnosis. The advent of MRI has decreased the use of myelography because MRI has better resolution, usually does not require the injection of contrast media and has no ionising radiation.

Side effects

Improper injection may cause spinal-cord inflammation (arachnoiditis) or may cause nerve-root injury or perforation of the annulus fibrosus (which can lead to disc herniation). Headaches, dizziness, nausea and vomiting are common side effects that subside with time. Neurotoxic effects of the contrast medium can cause meningitis-like symptoms including referred pain into the limbs, **hyperreflexia** and cerebral or central nervous system–related symptoms (seizures, central nervous system ischemia, and visual and auditory changes).

Fluoroscopy

Fluoroscopy is an imaging technique that uses X-rays to produce real-time moving images of the internal structures of the body using a fluoroscope. A fluoroscope consists of an X-ray source and a fluorescent screen with the patient placed between the two. Modern fluoroscopes connect the screen to an X-ray image intensifier and video camera that allows for recording and displaying of the image on a monitor. Fluoroscopy can be used to trace the passage of contrast media though the body. Doctors can also record the moving X-ray images on film or video. Most modern X-ray image intensifiers have a pulsed system that turns the radiation on and off at set intervals. Some also have a 'freeze-frame' feature that holds the last image on the monitor for the practitioner, significantly reducing the radiation exposure to the patient.

Fluoroscopy is no longer a commonly used procedure; however, it does have some attributes that can be very useful for certain specific procedures.

Reasons to have this test

Fluoroscopy is most commonly used during surgical or investigative procedures. Orthopaedic procedures such as aligning a broken bone.

Other less common uses include orthopaedic evaluation of joint motion and blood flow studies (it can display blood flow to and from organs). A discogram image is made using fluoroscopy to guide a needle to an intervertebral disc where a radiologically visible dye is injected.

Reasons you might not be able to have this test
There are no **absolute contraindications**. Pregnancy is a relative contra-indication due to the risk to the developing embryo. Possible side effects include birth defects (for pregnant women) and cancer, due to radiation exposure.

Positive attributes
Fluoroscopy can be an invaluable tool due to its capacity to provide real-time images of the internal structures of the body, which can be viewed on a monitor and recorded during a medical procedure.

Negative attributes
Fluoroscopy uses high doses of ionising radiation compared to standard plain X-ray. Complicated fluoroscopic procedures often require longer exposure time, which gives a greater radiation dose to the patient. Anyone working within a two-metre radius of the fluoroscope must be protected by lead shielding (lead apron, lead gloves, lead eyeglasses and so on), which can be heavy or cumbersome.

Side effects
Possible hair loss (alopecia). Increased risk of cancer, which is directly pro-portional to the radiation dose. The risk of radiation burns to the skin (erythema) are virtually non-existent below a certain threshold of radia-tion dose, but nearly 100 per cent at dose levels significantly higher than this threshold. Radiation burns are uncommon in standard fluoroscopic procedures.

Discography

Discography is an X-ray imaging technique that evaluates the integrity of the intervertebral disc. It involves the injecting of water-soluble contrast material into the centre of the intervertebral disc. The test determines whether an intervertebral disc is painful and whether it is the source of the patient's low back pain. As a test it has a very high specificity rating, which means that when this test is positive it can be relied on to identify the presence of a painful disc. The main feature of this investigation is that it tests a patient's response to disc stimulation directly. Discography is very rarely painful in asymptomatic patients, even those with degenerated discs, but is frequently positive (painful) in patients with low back pain. Therefore, discography determines whether a degenerative disc has become symptomatic. For the test to be positive, the injection must reproduce the patient's pain. Strikingly, many lumbar discs that are painful with discography show no external signs of damage or degeneration; they often appear normal and show no signs of herniation or prolapse on scans. Surgery is contraindicated for patients with a positive discogram in a disc that appears structurally normal. Discography is an especially useful test when other diagnostic procedures have failed to identify the source of back pain.

Reasons to have this test

Discography is indicated in cases where the exact source of back pain needs to be identified, such as those with persistent, severe symptoms when other diagnostic tests have failed to clearly confirm a suspected disc as the source of pain. Discography is a useful pre-surgical assessment used to confirm that the disc being operated on is the actual cause of the patient's back pain. It is also used for the assessment of patients in whom previous back surgery has failed.

Reasons you might not be able to have this test

Patients with a known bleeding disorder and those on anticoagulation therapy (blood-thinning medicine) may not be able to have this test. Those with a systemic infection or skin infection over the puncture site may not be able to have discography. This test may not be suitable for patients with severe spinal wear and tear. Severe spinal canal compromise at the disc level to be investigated. Psychiatric conditions such as post-traumatic stress disorder or schizophrenia can make the patient feel stressed with this procedure. Pregnancy and allergy to contrast dye are other patient conditions not suited to discography.

Positive attributes

Discography is currently the only reliable diagnostic test that can identify the disc as a pain generator. Failing to find a painful disc on discography should exclude surgery; so too should finding multiple painful discs or obtaining indeterminate results. Unwarranted back surgery can be prevented by heeding indeterminate or negative results. The results of a discogram help to confirm the need for surgery, which will increase the likelihood of a positive outcome from surgery. In cases with individuals who have had previous lumbar fusion, CT scans or MRI images are often distorted by the metal artefacts left in the patient, thus making discography the technique of choice in such cases.

Negative attributes

Fluoroscopy is required in order to guide the needle into the disc and a CT scan is required to image the area post-injection, both of which have ionising radiation. Discograms do not show the bones or nerves very well and do not show muscles. Few radiologists still perform this test, thus it may be difficult to find an imaging centre that offers this service. Some experts argue that discography is simply an 'informational tool' for the purpose of establishing a diagnosis for which no proven therapy exists.

Side effects

Infection of the disc called discitis sometimes occurs. The incidence of discitis is 2 to 3 per cent when a single-needle technique is used and 0.7 per cent when a double-needle technique is used. The occurrence of discitis becomes very rare when antibiotics are used after the procedure. Other possible side effects include spinal headache, infection, nerve damage, bleeding, disc injury, allergic reaction, nausea, seizures and increased pain.

Nuclear medicine

Nuclear medicine techniques employ radioactive tracer agents (radiopharmaceuticals) that are placed into the body through ingestion, inhalation or injection. Once in the body, the radioactive drug emits gamma rays that are picked up by a detector and converted into electrical signals that are processed by a computer to produce an image. Gamma rays have high energy, meaning most of them pass through the body, allowing for the production of accurate images. The intensity, symmetry and other characteristics captured on an image are then evaluated by a radiologist.

Currently there are several nuclear medicine techniques, such as scintigraphy, positron emission tomography (PET scan), single photon emission computed tomography (SPECT), super scan and three-phase bone scan. New technologies and procedures are constantly being developed and old ones are refined. Bone scans (scintigraphy) are presently the most frequently ordered nuclear medicine procedure, accounting for over half the studies performed in a nuclear medicine department. SPECT imaging is a newer form of 3-D bone scan that uses one or multiple cameras.

Currently the most commonly used radiopharmaceuticals are a family of drugs called diphosphonates, which have faster blood clearance and higher skeletal uptake than previous generations of radiopharmaceuticals.

Bone scan

Reasons to have this test
Bone scans provide valuable information when clinical findings are compelling but plain films are negative or equivocal. Bone-scanning techniques are useful for the evaluation of soft tissue, bone and joint disorders. Any disorder that decreases or increases blood flow or bone cell activity or both will result in an abnormal image. SPECT imaging is useful for the detection of tumours, symptomatic spondylolysis, facet-joint pain and pseudo-arthrosis following spinal fusion. Bone scans are very useful in finding areas of high bone turnover, which happens in new fractures, some arthritic conditions and certain tumours.

Reasons you might not be able to have this test
Dehydration is an absolute contraindication. For those on dialysis, radiopharmaceutical injection should be performed before dialysis. Pregnancy is a relative contraindication because of the risk of transmission of radiopharmaceuticals to the developing foetus. If a bone scan is performed on a breastfeeding mother, her breast milk will carry some of the drug for several days after the procedure. Formula feeding is recommended during this time.

Positive attributes

Bone scanning is a very sensitive examination. Bone scans provide a distinct advantage of being able to identify physiologic and metabolic changes in the body days or even weeks before gross structural changes caused by disease are detectable. An example of this is a stress fracture in the tibia (shin) that is forming but is not yet identifiable on X-ray—this sort of fracture will often show up on a bone scan first. This can allow for early diagnosis and treatment, which can often help patients get better faster. SPECT enables radiologists to view areas in a 3-D format that greatly enhances their ability to accurately localise and identify a wide range of structural problems.

Negative attributes

Bone scans involve the use of ionising radiation, so overuse or inappropriate use of bone scan should be avoided. Although it provides a high degree of sensitivity, bone scanning lacks the ability to provide anatomical specificity. To accommodate this shortfall, X-rays, CT or MRI are often ordered in conjunction with bone scanning.

Side effects

There is a radiation dose absorbed by the body; the exact amount absorbed by the patient is dependent on a number of factors such as organ pathology, tracer distribution and kidney health. The radiation dose absorbed in a whole body bone scan is approximately 20 to 30 times less than a standard lumbar CT scan procedure.

Bone densitometry

Bone densiometry is the study of bone mineral density (BMD). Several techniques measure BMD, such as conventional radiography, quantitative CT (QCT), single-photon absorptiometry (SPA), dual-photon absorptiometry (DPA), quantitative ultrasonography (QUS), and dual-energy X-ray absorptiometry (DEXA). Bone densiometry is used to diagnose osteoporosis and osteopaenia (bone-weakening disorders); currently DEXA is the established gold standard for bone-density testing. Bone-mineral density is defined by the T-score. This is calculated based on the peak bone mass that occurs between 20 and 35 years of age. T-scores of between –1.0 and –2.5 constitute mild bone weakness (osteopenia) and scores greater than –2.5 constitute substantial bone loss (osteoporosis). The Z-score is another standard reference used to evaluate BMD and is based on the level of bone loss of a patient compared to the bone density of a healthy person of the same age.

DEXA employs the use of two X-ray beams of different energy levels, which are measured as they passed through the body. The number of X-rays that pass through the body provides a bone-mineral density score. A DEXA scan normally takes between 10 and 30 minutes to complete. The hip and lumbar spine are the two most commonly assessed sites using DEXA; however, other sites such as the lower radius in the forearm are also used.

Heel ultrasound is another method of measuring BMD, although it is not currently standardised and has poor correlation with other BMD scans. An advantage of heel ultrasound is that it does not involve any ionising radiation. The major disadvantage is that it is not nearly as precise at measuring BMD as a DEXA.

Over a lifetime women have a one in four chance of developing an osteoporotic fracture, while men have a one in eight chance. Complications from a fracture in geriatric patients results in increased mortality rates. A third of men with osteoporotic hip fractures die within one year of fracture and nearly one-fifth of women in the same situation die. The risk of fracture decreases as BMD increases, thus early detection of decreased bone density can be lifesaving.

Pregnant women are at risk of diminished BMD in the first two trimesters. This is due to the foetus using the mother's calcium and phosphate stores for development. DEXA may be helpful in assessing pregnant women for their risk of fracture related to weight and posture changes and decreased BMD.

Children are more difficult to evaluate because T-scores are based on adult bone-mineral density. The Z-score, which measures the mean BMD of matched age individuals is used instead. However, assessment is not that simple. Z-scores do not take into account normal bone-mass changes with age, pubertal stage and gender, so appropriate reference standards must be used.

DEXA

Reasons to have this test
This is useful for women over the age of 65 and men over the age of 70. At-risk patients such as those with a prior history of fracture, low dietary calcium, low vitamin D levels, use of corticosteroid drugs, smoking, excess alcohol intake, rheumatoid arthritis, history of parental hip fracture, chronic kidney and liver disease, chronic respiratory disease, long-term use of phenobarbital or phenytoin medications, gastrointestinal disease, sedentary lifestyle, hyperprolactinemia and hypercorticalism. DEXA is also used to monitor treatment of osteoporosis.

Reasons you might not be able to have this test
Scanning within a week of other radiological procedures requiring contrast or nuclear medicine–based investigations is contraindicated. If the person's weight is greater than 120 kilograms, it is a relative contraindication as some large individuals may not fit into the DEXA scanner machine. There is also a relative contraindication for women who are (or may be) pregnant.

Positive attributes
The radiation doses used in DEXA are very low (10 per cent of a chest X-ray). Due to the low radiation dose, technicians can often remain in the same room during the procedure without the need for lead shielding. DEXA is fast, precise, inexpensive and widely available. DEXA can be used during pregnancy if clinically indicated. DEXA has the added advantage over other bone-density testing of being able to evaluate body composition (fat versus lean mass).

Negative attributes
DEXA cannot accommodate large individuals weighing over 120 kilograms; limb analysis may be done instead. Bilateral hip replacements or bilateral hip pins or screws would prevent the hip sites from being scanned. Similarly, metallic rods or spinal fusion devices in the lumbar spine would rule out scanning at this site. In older patients lumbar scans can produce misleading results due to the presence of **osteophytes** (arthritic bony

spurs), which artificially increase the BMD. DEXA has distorted results based on skeletal size. Larger-sized individuals can have an overestimated T-scores, while petite individuals have underestimated scores. DEXA cannot establish the cause of low BMD.

Side effects
There is some ionising radiation absorbed by the body.

Ultrasonography

Ultrasound (ultrasonography) is a diagnostic technology that uses high frequency sound (ultrasound) to form a two-dimensional image used for the examination and measurement of internal body structures and the detection of bodily abnormalities. Ultrasound works by sending sound pulses into your body using a probe. The sound waves travel into your body until they hit boundaries between tissues (that is, soft tissue and bone). Some sound waves get reflected back to the probe, while some continue on until they hit a boundary and are reflected. The distance the reflected waves travel is calculated by the machine's processor to form a two-dimensional image that is displayed on a screen. Ultrasound is used to view muscles, tendons and many internal organs, capturing their size, position, structure and any pathological lesion in real-time images. There are two other forms of ultrasound currently in use: 3-D ultrasound imaging and Doppler ultrasound. 3-D ultrasound simply takes several 2-D scans and combines them by using specialised computer software to produce a 3-D image. Doppler ultrasound is useful in measuring blood flow.

Reason to have this test
Arthritic conditions, soft-tissue lesions, internal derangement of joints, infection and examination of some hollow organs such as in-utero examination.

Reasons you might not be able to have this test
Currently there are no known contraindications to patients who have diagnostic ultrasound. The long-term effects of ultrasound exposure at diagnostic levels are still unknown.

Positive attributes

Ultrasound is relatively inexpensive compared to other imaging techniques such a MRI. Ultrasound produces real-time images which can be viewed on a monitor by both the practitioner/technician and the patient, and the probe can be moved or angled to obtain various views. Ultrasound can reveal joint lesions in the early stages of a disease as well as in patients who only report pain.

Negative attributes

Ultrasonography does have some potential side effects: it enhances inflammatory response and can cause excessive heat in soft tissues. The images generated by this technology are of relatively low resolution and are best read as moving images while being recorded, rather than as still images after they have been printed.

Nerve block

A nerve block is an invasive medical procedure to relieve pain by interfering with nerve signals to the brain. The procedure involves the injection of a substance onto or around a suspected pain-transmitting nerve that effectively blocks pain signals to the brain. Depending on the substance used, nerve blocks can either provide short-term or long-term effects. Short-term nerve blocks often use a local anaesthetic, but they can be accompanied by other substances such as a corticosteroid to reduce inflammation or painkillers such as opioids. Long-term nerve blocks (sometimes called permanent nerve blocks) use substances such as alcohol or phenol to selectively destroy nerve tissue, which may provide long-term pain relief.

Nerve blocks are commonly used diagnostically to determine the source of pain, treat painful conditions, as a short-term relief after a medical procedure or as an anaesthetic for simple surgical procedures. Nerve blocks are often used when conventional pain-relieving drugs fail to provide adequate relief or the patient has bad side effects from such drugs. Often a test nerve block using local anaesthetic is done prior to the procedure to evaluate the effectiveness of the procedure. If a patient has good pain relief with the local anaesthetic, the doctor may then inject a longer acting nerve block agent.

Imaging guidance such as ultrasound, fluoroscopy or CT is often used to help the doctor guide the needle to the precise location so that the procedure has maximal benefit and minimal complications.

Diagnostic lumbar facet joint–nerve blocks are relatively safe, valid and reliable. There is strong evidence for the diagnostic accuracy of lumbar facet joint–nerve blocks in evaluating spinal pain.

Reasons to have this test

Patients with acute or chronic pain that are unresponsive to conservative care benefit from this procedure. It can be used as a diagnostic procedure to evaluate potential sources of pain. Others who can also benefit are those with complex regional pain syndrome, coccydynia, phantom pain after amputation, lingering pain after an attack of shingles or nerve pain due to frostbite.

Reasons you might not be able to have this test

Patients with blood-clotting diseases or those on blood-thinning medication (such as Heparin or Warfarin). Patients with a bowel obstruction or current infection.

Positive attributes

The procedure is relatively safe and patients can often return to normal activities the next day. The procedure is usually done under local anaesthetic, removing the need for a general anaesthetic, which has more risks.

Negative attributes

Risk of complications include: paralysis, damage to arteries that supply blood to the spinal cord, hypotension (low blood pressure), accidental injection into an artery, lung puncture, damage to the kidneys, diarrhoea, allergic reactions, increased pain and weakness in the legs.

Recommendations

As a therapeutic procedure this should be used only after more conservative treatments have failed. Patients should only agree to have a nerve block performed under imaging guidance to minimise the chance of complications.

Electrodiagnostic tests

There are several forms of electrodiagnostic testing; the two most common are nerve conductions studies (NCS) and electromyograms (EMG).

NCS measure how well and how fast the nerves can send electrical signals. Small electrodes are strategically placed on the patient's skin, a shock-emitting electrode is placed over the nerve and a recording electrode is placed over a muscle controlled by that nerve. Several quick electrical pulses are given to the nerve and then the time it takes the muscle to contract is measured. The speed of the response is called the conduction velocity. The same nerves on the other side of the body may be studied for comparison. NCS are usually done before an EMG if both tests have been ordered. NCS may take from 15 minutes to one hour or more, depending on how many nerves and muscles are studied.

NCS may be accompanied by an electromyogram (also known as needle EMG), which involves the use of fine needles placed within a muscle to measure its electrical output. A needle electrode attached by wires to a recording machine is inserted into a specific muscle to be tested. The needle has a microscopic electrode that picks up both the normal and abnormal electrical signals given off by a muscle. Once in place, the electrical activity of the resting muscle is measured. The doctor will then ask the patient to slowly and steadily contract the muscle. This electrical activity is measured. The needle may be moved several times to record the activity of the muscle in different parts of the muscle. The activity of the muscle is displayed as wavy and spiky lines on a video monitor, which can be recorded, or may be heard on a loudspeaker as machine gun–like popping sounds when the muscle contracts. An EMG generally takes between 30 and 60 minutes.

If a patient is experiencing leg pain or numbness, they may have these tests to find out to what extent the nerves themselves are affected. These tests check how well the spinal nerves and the nerves in a patient's arms and legs are working. These are invaluable tests for assessing the damage or dysfunction to neurological structures that cannot be detected through routine neurological examination. The test is typically performed by a neurologist.

Nerve conduction studies

Reasons to have this test
This covers any condition involving symptoms such as numbness, pins and needles, weakness or pain. That includes a herniated disc with neural compression, **spinal stenosis**, spinal cord lesion and neurological pathology.

Reasons you might not be able to have this test
Currently there are no known contraindications.

Positive attributes
NCS have been found to be safe for individuals with pacemakers. NCS can help localise the site or level of the problem if it's neurologically based. The test can be performed at an outpatient clinic. Nerve-conduction studies can be used to monitor nerve function over time to determine disease progression or resolution. It can also assess complications of treatment (for example, chemotherapy), as well as identifying the disease course.

Negative attributes
The test is mildly painful during the testing procedure. Often other diagnostic tests are required to figure out the exact nature of the problem.

Complications
There are no known risks involved with NCS.

Recommendations
A patient should not smoke for three hours before the test, and should avoid eating or drinking foods that contain caffeine (such as coffee, tea, cola and chocolate) for three hours before the test. Patients should wear loose-fitting clothing so muscles and nerves can be easily tested. You may be given a hospital gown to wear. On the morning of the test, patients should thoroughly clean the extremities to be tested with soap and water. Patients should not apply oil, lotion or cream to the extremities to be tested. Patients need to advise the neurologist if they have a pacemaker.

Electromyogram

Reasons to have this test
Patients with nerve root or nerve plexus problems. Nerve disorders such as an entrapped nerve or disorders that affect the nervous system such as diabetes. Muscle disorders (muscular dystrophy), or neuromuscular junction disorders such as myasthenia gravis.

Reasons you might not be able to have this test
An implantable cardioverter-defibrillator device (ICD) can't be exposed to this treatment, but a pacemaker is acceptable. Bleeding disorders and those on blood-thinning medications cannot participate.

Positive attributes
An EMG is very safe; it can be performed in a doctor's office.

Negative attributes
There is a very small risk of infection due to the use of fine-needle electrodes. The test can be mildly painful during needle insertion as well as during the testing procedure. Often other diagnostic tests are required to figure out the exact nature of the problem.

Complications
Infection due to the introduction of pathogen through the skin during needle insertion is a risk. Needle insertion may produce some minor bruising at the skin and muscle level.

Recommendations
A patient should not smoke for three hours before the test. It's best for a patient not to eat or drink foods that contain caffeine (such as coffee, tea, cola and chocolate) for three hours before the test. Patients should wear loose-fitting clothing so muscles and nerves can be tested. You may be given a hospital gown to wear. On the morning of the test, thoroughly clean the extremities to be tested with soap and water. Do not apply oil, lotion or cream to the extremities to be tested. Advise the neurologist if you have a pacemaker.

Conclusion

With the ever-expanding array of imaging and diagnostic methods available, selection of what's appropriate can be daunting and confusing to both practitioners and patients. It is important that the patient and practitioner work together to select the most appropriate steps for the patient's unique set of circumstances and condition. Failure to do so can result in inappropriate diagnostic tests being ordered, adverse effects from the diagnostic procedure, or simply making the patient feel excluded from the decision-making process.

Studies estimate that up to two-thirds of spinal CT scans and MRI may be inappropriate. One problem with inappropriate imaging is that it may result in findings that are distracting, irrelevant and unnecessarily alarming. Furthermore, one study showed that surgery rates are highest where imaging rates are highest. There is also a trend toward more surgery and higher costs among patients who have an MRI earlier in their treatment compared to those only having X-rays. However, no association is shown with having a better end result.

Based on this information, one can begin to understand the complexities of surrounding back pain and its diagnosis. Imaging and other diagnostic procedures are clinically important and may be necessary in order to rule out specific diagnostic possibilities. However, these must be ordered judiciously and should only be prescribed once a thorough risk–benefit assessment has been considered, and all parties are in agreement on the chosen path to take.

4 Treatment

Back treatments

Despite the fact that back pain is one of the most common musculoskeletal disorders, consensus regarding its management has not been reached. Although most cases of acute low back pain are self-limiting and spontaneously resolve within several weeks, there is a proportion of these cases that will fail to resolve and become chronic back pain. The good news is that there are many treatment options for those suffering with back pain. The bad news is that it can be difficult to know which treatment will work best for you or whether the treatment is effective.

Although there have been many advances in treatment for back pain over the past several decades, the effectiveness of some of these procedures remains a concern. About one fifth of patients are still in pain after surgery, and almost as many who have discectomy develop failed back surgery syndrome (see Chapter 2). A more positive aspect of back pain is that approximately 85 per cent of chronic low back pain is mechanical, meaning it is not due to neurological or disease involvement. Unfortunately, mechanical back pain is one of the most difficult musculoskeletal problems to effectively diagnose and treat.

Presently there are so many treatments, therapies and rehabilitation options that it is nearly impossible for the average person to figure out the most appropriate one for their particular problem.

This chapter aims to highlight some of the more commonly used and effective therapies currently available for the treatment of back pain. We have provided a brief description of each therapy, listed the positive and negative attributes of each treatment and identified the potential risks and complications. What is presented here is not all-encompassing, as there are new treatments and therapies being developed all the time.

Invasive therapies involve penetrating the skin, such as open surgeries. Other than in emergency situations, invasive procedures are reserved for situations where more conservative approaches have failed. Non-invasive therapies are generally safer than surgery, less expensive and typically do not require a period of rehabilitation immediately afterwards.

Non-invasive therapies

Dozens of different types of non-invasive therapies have been developed. Some, such as acupuncture and manipulation are thousands of years old. The difficulty often faced by back pain sufferers is deciding which non-invasive therapy to try or to try next. Which therapy is right for you? Despite all we know about back pain, there are no clear prediction rules to answer this question. What we are left with is the best advice of the clinicians we seek care from. Clinicians are not exposed to every possible therapy, and they are influenced by personal experience and patient reports. Clinicians can only give you their opinion of the options available to you and the relative merits of these options.

Of the many alternatives to standard or western medical approaches, here are a few:

- Acupuncture and dry needling
- Advice to stay active or rest
- Cryotherapy (cold therapy) and thermotherapy (heat therapy)
- Electrical muscle stimulation
- Exercise therapy
- Interferential current
- Kinesiology taping
- Massage therapy
- Myofascial release (ART, fascial manipulation, Guā Shā, Graston technique)
- Spinal manipulative therapy (SMT)
- TENS and PENS
- Therapeutic ultrasound

- Traction therapy
- Trigger point therapy

Acupuncture and dry needling

Acupuncture originated in China and has been used in Asian cultures for millennia, since the Han dynasty. It is a form of traditional Chinese medicine. It was first described in the medical compilation *Huangdi Neijing* (*Yellow Emperor's Inner Classic*), dating from 200 BC to 200 AD. The Chinese word for acupuncture, *zhen jiu,* means 'needling burning'. Acupuncture has shown a steady increase in popularity in western cultures over the past few decades.

Acupuncture is widely used in healthcare systems in many countries in Asia; it is officially recognised by governments and well-received by the general public. Acupuncture is defined as the placement of fine needles at anatomically defined sites of the body (acupuncture points) or sensitive spots (*ah shi* points) for therapeutic purposes. These points lie along meridian lines, which are believed to govern energy flow (called Qi) through the body in traditional eastern philosophy. The aim of acupuncture is to balance these energy flows.

There are a few different acupuncture techniques of needle stimulation including needle thrusting, twisting or rotating, or electrical stimulation to achieve different treatment effects. There are also some acupuncture-related therapies such as laser acupuncture, injections into acupuncture points and acupressure that are commonly used in clinical settings. Acupuncture also includes moxibustion—the burning of selected herbs on or over the skin.

Dry needling is a fairly broad term used to differentiate 'non-injection' needling from medical 'injection needling', which involves the use of a hypodermic syringe and an injectable agent, such as saline or an anaesthetic. Dry needling involves the use of solid, fine filament needles, similar to those used in acupuncture, and it relies on the stimulation of target tissue to create specific reactions for its therapeutic effect.

Deep dry needling for treating trigger points was first introduced by Czech physician Karel Lewit in 1979. Unlike acupuncture, dry needling does not use acupuncture points or meridians to figure out the placement of the needle. Dry needling for the treatment of myofascial trigger points is based on theories similar, but not exclusive, to traditional acupuncture. Dry needling is strictly based on western medicine principles and is increasingly used in the management of musculoskeletal and sports injuries. Originally, dry needling was restricted to placement within a myofascial trigger point; however, in the 1980s it was expanded to use on other soft-tissue structures of the body. In 2005 another form of dry needling was developed called superficial dry needling. It is similar to traditional dry needling except the needle is only inserted approximately 5 mm to 10 mm into the tissue superficial to the trigger point. Technically both acupuncture and dry needling can be considered invasive because they break the skin barrier. Acupressure, by contrast, does not break the skin and is considered non-invasive.

Reasons to have this treatment (in western medicine)
Acute and chronic pain, muscle spasm, soft tissue strain or sprain, hypermobility, trigger point syndrome, tendinopathies, bursitis, capsulitis, facet joint irritation, degenerative disc disease, muscle hypertonicity, myofascial adhesions and scar tissue.

Reasons this treatment might not be suitable for you
Absolute contraindications include medical emergencies (such as cardiac arrest), allergies to metals, needling at sites of active infection or skin lesions, lymphoedema, malignant tumours or the abdomen of pregnant females. Electro-acupuncture should not be applied across the spinal cord and is contraindicated for patients with a cardiac pacemaker. Relative contraindications include naturally occurring haemorrhagic diseases (for example, haemophilia), patients on high levels of blood-thinning medications (in which case, finer gauge needles must be used). Epilepsy and diabetes are also contraindications. Pregnant patients should be cautious, as needling certain acupuncture points may cause strong uterine contractions and can induce labour.

Prohibited areas of needling include nipples, external genitalia, the umbilicus and the eyeball.

Treatment effects
Acupuncture can induce **analgesia**, protect the body against infections, and regulate various bodily functions.

Positive attributes

Needling is safe if it is performed properly by a well-trained practitioner. Advantages of needling are that it is simple, convenient and has few contra-indications. In many developing countries, where medical personnel and medicines are still lacking, the proper use of this simple and economic therapy benefits a large number of patients.

Negative attributes

Treatment can be uncomfortable or even painful for some patients. Some patients have a fear of needles and may not be able to tolerate treatment.

Side effects

Common adverse effects include post-treatment soreness. Less common adverse effects include bruising due to perforation of a blood vessel. During treatment, some patients may feel faint, light-headed or nauseous. Pain during needle insertion is not uncommon, particularly in highly sensitive individuals. However, skilful and rapid penetration of the needle through the skin is usually painless. Rare complications include pneumothorax (perforated lung) and infection. Rarely needles can break, which is often due to poor-quality needle manufacturing, erosion between the shaft and the handle of the needle, strong muscle spasm or sudden movement by the patient, or incorrect withdrawal of a stuck or bent needle. If a broken needle becomes completely embedded under the skin, surgical removal of the needle may be necessary.

Recommendations

Caution should be used on pregnant patients, as certain acupuncture points may induce labour. Before starting treatment, all potential risks should be outlined to you, and all your questions answered prior to your giving consent. Special care must be taken with patients with blood diseases and practitioners must wear protective gloves. The skin should be examined to ensure that it is clean prior to treatment.

If a patient begins to display adverse symptoms such as light-headedness, nausea or faintness from needling, the needles should be removed immediately and the patient should be made to lie flat on their back with the head down and legs raised, as symptoms are usually short-lived due to insufficient blood supply to the brain. A fruit drink or something sweet to eat often helps with these symptoms, which usually disappear after a short rest. In severe cases, first aid should be given and the patient should be taken to the hospital for examination.

Proof of effectiveness

Acupuncture provides a short-term clinically relevant effect. It can be effective in managing patients with low back pain, particularly patients with positive expectations about acupuncture, which suggests a psychological element. Patients treated with dry needling in addition to a standard therapy regimen have been found to have clear and significantly better outcomes compared to standard therapy only.

Advice to stay active or rest

In the past practitioners often advised patients suffering from low back pain to rest. The term 'rest' varied, but generally implied remaining in bed for the entire day, only getting out to use the toilet or feed oneself. In the 1980s and '90s new research emerged that indicated that bed rest resulted in negative effects such as muscle thinning, de-conditioning and deterioration of many body functions. A change occurred by end of the millennium, when practitioners began to shift their thinking to have patients be more active in order to better manage their low back pain. Current studies show that advice to stay active is more effective than bed rest for people with acute low back pain. However, in the short term there may be little or no difference between staying active and bed rest for patients with sciatica. The national clinical guidelines from at least 11 countries on acute low back pain agree on the need to reassure patients, promote early and progressive physical activation, and discourage bed rest.

Recommendations

When you seek professional help for your back pain, be wary of advice to rest for more than a day or two, especially bed rest. Typically practitioners who do not keep up with current clinical guidelines and research findings give outdated recommendations, such as bed rest for low back pain.

Cryotherapy and thermotherapy

Cryotherapy: Cold therapy is defined as the therapeutic application of any substance to the body that removes heat from the body, resulting in decreased tissue temperature. As with thermotherapy (heat therapy), cryotherapy has been used as a therapeutic treatment for thousands of years, but it is not until recently that we have begun to better understand its application.

Traditionally ice has been recommended for acute injury treatment. Temperature changes within the body are dependent on several variables such as the method of application, duration of application, initial temperature and depth of subcutaneous fat. The therapeutic range when cooling soft tissue is a target tissue temperature reduction of 10°C to 15°C.

Cryotherapy can be applied to the body via conduction (cold packs, ice massage, cryopressure garments combining cold with compression), convection (cold whirlpool immersion, contrast baths) or evaporation (vapocoolant sprays).

Reasons to have this treatment
Cryotherapy is useful in the management of acute and chronic pain, oedema and inflammation; to enhance movement; and to decrease muscle spasms.

Reasons this treatment might not be suitable for you
Avoid treating areas of impaired sensation, impaired circulation, peripheral vascular disease, over-regenerating peripheral nerves, deep or open wounds, angina pectoris, severe cardiac disease, cold hypersensitivity (such as Raynaud's disease), hives, rash and cold haemoglobinuria.

Treatment
Cryotherapy decreases pain receptor input and pain perception, inflammation, local metabolic rate, tissue extensibility, muscle spasm, nerve-signalling speed and circulation, and induces local constriction of blood vessels.

Positive attributes
Cryotherapy decreases tissue blood flow by causing constricted blood vessels and reduces tissue metabolism, oxygen utilisation, inflammation

and muscle spasm. Cold therapy is easily available, can be used at home, is relatively inexpensive and safe, and, when effective, can provide some immediate and obvious relief.

Negative attributes
Frostbite can occur if proper safety precautions are not followed. Reflexes and motor function are impaired after treatment for up to 30 minutes.

Side effects
Bradycardia (decreased heart rate), Raynaud's disease, hives, cold erythema (rash), cold haemoglobinuria, frostbite, neuropathy and slowed wound healing due to decreased metabolic activity.

Recommendations
Care should be taken when applying cold therapy if you have high blood pressure, as constricting blood vessels can increase blood pressure. Care should be taken when applying cryotherapy on an area where nerves pass close to the surface (such as near the elbow). Use short treatment times (for example, 10-minute applications followed by 30-minute rest periods), rather than long or continuous treatment, as this has been shown to provide better results. It has the added benefit of allowing the skin temperature to return to normal while the deeper tissues remain cold.

Proof of effectiveness
There is still not enough evidence about the effect of the application of cold for low back pain of any duration. Contrast therapy, which alternates between heat and cold therapy, has been shown to provide no additional therapeutic benefits compared with heat or cold therapy used alone.

Thermotherapy: Heat therapy has been used since antiquity as a therapeutic treatment for many ailments including musculoskeletal injuries. Of the therapeutic agents used in ancient times, few are still commonly used today; thermotherapy has proven to be one such exception. Traditionally, heat is used for longer-term (chronic) injuries. Heat therapy is believed to increase circulation, enhance healing, increase soft-tissue extensibility and control pain. Heat therapy can be administered via conduction (hot packs, paraffin dips, microwavable grain-filled cloth bags or electric heating

Lateral core endurance test

For this test you will need a stopwatch and another person to function as an assessor.

1. Begin by lying down on an exercise mat on your left side, with both thighs together and both feet on the floor, the right foot placed just in front of the left. Maintain a slight bend at the waist.
2. Place the left elbow under the shoulder or just off centre in a comfortable position. Be sure to keep the outside (lateral) part of the weight-bearing forearm and hand in contact with the mat throughout the test.
3. Raise your torso off the mat by pushing yourself up so your weight is on your elbow, forearm and feet, forming a straight line from the shoulder down to the feet. Timing begins when the assessor deems you have stopped moving.
4. Hold this position for as long as you can. Timing stops when you can no longer hold the starting position. The person being assessed is allowed one warning from the assessor for a positional fault; time is stopped and the test is over if a second fault is committed.
5. Take at least a 60-second break, and then test the opposite side.

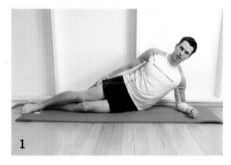 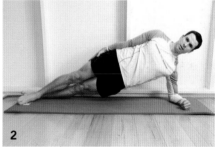

POSITIONAL FAULTS:
*   Failing to maintain a straight line from the shoulder to the foot (for example, dropping or sagging at the pelvis).
*   Rotating the upper shoulder forward or backward.

TIPS: Write down your times in a log book. Re-test every four to six weeks and compare the times to track your progress. When re-testing, try to have the same assessor, as different assessors may view faults differently.

CAUTIONS: Avoid this test if you are unable to achieve the starting position or cannot bear weight on your elbow or shoulder.

Anterior core endurance test

For this test you will need a stopwatch and another person to function as an assessor.

1. Start in a sit-up position, supported by an angled backrest (approximately 60 degrees).
2. Keep your feet firmly held down by either using toe straps or having an assessor hold them down with their hands.
3. Bend your knees and hips so that your legs form a 90 degree angle and your feet are flat on the mat. Fold your arms across your chest, grasping the opposite shoulder with your hands.
4. Timing begins when the assessor pulls the backrest 10 cm away from your back. Hold this position for as long as you can.
5. Timing stops when any part of your body touches the backrest. The person being assessed is allowed one warning from the assessor for a positional fault; time is stopped and the test is over if a second fault is committed.

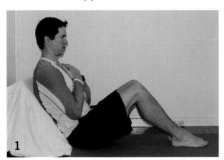 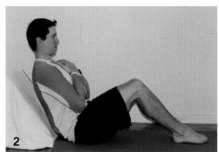

POSITIONAL FAULTS:
- Failing to hold the starting position.
- Flexing or extending any part of the spine into a position other than the starting position.
- An excessively increased arch in the back.

TIPS: Write down your times in a log book. Re-test every four to six weeks and compare the times to track your progress. When re-testing, try to have the same assessor, as different assessors may view faults differently.

CAUTIONS: Avoid this test if you are unable to achieve the starting position or cannot have pressure placed on top of your feet.

Posterior core endurance test

For this test you will need a stopwatch and another person to function as an assessor, as well as a sturdy, covered table (like a massage or chiropractic table) and a sturdy chair. Any firm table that will bear your weight, covered in a towel, can be used for this test.

1. Place the chair facing the table as shown in the pictures below.
2. Lie face-down on the table and slowly move yourself down the table towards the chair so the top half your body is held in a horizontal position off the table, but the top of the pelvis remains on the table. Support your upper body with the chair until the text begins (picture 1).
3. Make sure your feet, legs and pelvis are kept firmly held down on the table either by using feet straps or having your assessor hold your legs down with their hands.
4. If the assessor is holding your legs for the test, timing begins just before they hold your legs down. If you're using leg straps, timing begins when you remove your hands from the support chair and cross them over your chest. Hold this position for as long as you can.
5. Timing stops when you drop from the horizontal position or require the support of the chair. The person being assessed is allowed one warning from the assessor for a positional fault; time is stopped and the test is over if a second fault is committed.

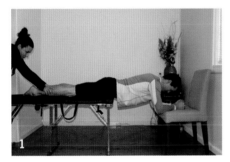 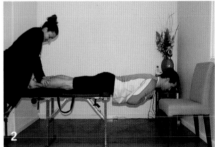

POSITIONAL FAULTS:
• Failing to maintain a straight line from the shoulder to the foot (for example, dropping or sagging at the pelvis).

TIPS: Write down you times in a log book. Re-test every four to six weeks and compare the times to track your progress. When re-testing, try to have the same assessor, as different assessors may view faults differently.

CAUTIONS: Avoid this test if you are unable to achieve the starting position or you cannot have pressure placed across the back of your legs or feet.

Abdominal bracing

1. Begin flat on your back with your legs bent so that your feet are flat on the floor at a comfortable angle.
2. Lightly place both hands either side of your navel, about 5 cm apart, palms down, fingers pointing inwards. This will allow you to feel when and if your core muscles are contracting. However, it is not necessary to hold this position throughout the exercise.
3. Perform abdominal bracing by contracting all your tummy muscles and low back muscles. Imagine the way you would tense up if you were about to be punched in the stomach. (Another way of describing it is to bear down as though you are trying to defecate.) You should feel the muscles under your hands contract, become hard and spring up towards your fingers.
4. Hold the abdominal bracing for two seconds, then relax. Rest for 2 seconds then repeat.
5. Perform 2 sets of 10 reps. Rest for 60 seconds between sets.

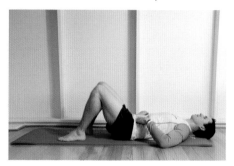

Intermediate version: If you wish to increase the difficulty of this exercise, change steps 4 and 5 so you hold the abdominal bracing for ten seconds, rest for five seconds, then repeat. Perform two sets of four reps. Rest for 60 seconds between sets.

TIPS: Avoid contracting too forcefully and holding your breath. Do not flex your neck or push your back down into the mat in an attempt to flatten your lower back.

Primary muscles worked: Rectus abdominis, external and internal obliques, transversus abdominis and pelvic floor.

CAUTIONS: Avoid this exercise if you have a hernia or an abdominal aortic aneurysm. Immediately stop the exercise if for any reason you experience pain while performing it.

Side bridge: remedial

1. Begin by standing with your right side parallel to a sturdy, flat wall, approximately one outstretched arm's length away.
2. Place your left leg slightly in front of the right.
3. Bend the right elbow to 90 degrees and place your forearm on the wall, parallel to the floor, at about shoulder height (see picture 1). Maintain a rigid torso and keep your body in a straight line when leaning against the wall.
4. Perform abdominal bracing.
5. Slowly twist your body by pivoting your feet until you are facing the wall with both forearms along the wall and your feet pointing at the wall (see picture 2).
6. Pause for one second, then continue to pivot your feet and twist your entire body (not just your spine) until your left forearm is along the wall and you are facing the opposite direction to the starting point.
7. Repeat steps 3–6 for two sets of five reps. Rest for 60 seconds between sets.

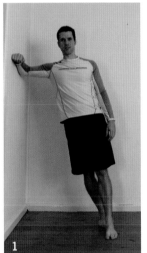 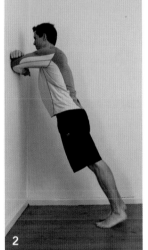 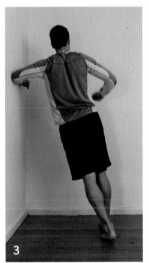

TIPS: Keep your torso rigid and in a straight line. Only perform this exercise on a non-slip surface.

Primary muscles worked: Internal and external obliques, and the quadratus lumborum.

CAUTIONS: Avoid this exercise if you are unable to bear weight on your elbows, forearms or shoulders. Do not perform this exercise against an unstable surface, or against a wall that will not support your body weight.

Half side bridge

1. Begin by lying down on your left side on an exercise mat with your thighs stacked on top of each other, knees bent to 90 degrees and both feet on the mat, with the right foot placed in front of the left. Start with your knees bent and your feet placed 20–30 cm in front of your hips.
2. Place your left elbow under the shoulder or just slightly to the side in a comfortable position.
3. Keep the outside (lateral) part of your left forearm and hand in contact with the mat throughout the exercise.
4. Perform abdominal bracing.
5. Push your hips forward until you are no longer bent at the waist, and simultaneously push up onto your left elbow and forearm so that your entire torso is off the mat.
6. Hold this position while abdominal bracing for 10 seconds.
7. Slowly lower yourself back down to the start position by bending at the waist.
8. Rest for five seconds, then repeat steps 4–8. Perform two sets of four reps on each side. Rest for 60 seconds between sets.

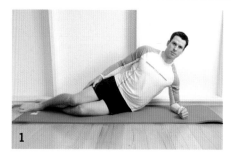 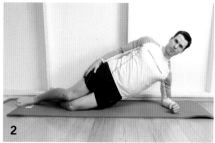

TIPS: Keep your torso rigid and in a straight line, and don't allow your pelvis to drop down. Avoid letting your knees separate. Swap sides every two sets to allow each side to rest.

Primary muscles worked: Internal and external obliques, and the quadratus lumborum.

CAUTIONS: Avoid this exercise if you are unable to bear weight on your shoulders, elbows or forearms, wrist or lateral thighs.

Side bridge

1. Begin by lying down on your left side on an exercise mat with your thighs and knees together and both feet on the mat, with the right foot placed in front of the left. Start with your knees bent and your feet 20–30 cm in front of your hips so you are bent at the waist.
2. Place your left elbow under the shoulder or just to the side in a comfortable position.
3. Keep the outside (lateral) part of your left forearm and hand in contact with the mat throughout the exercise.
4. Perform abdominal bracing.
5. Push your hips forward until you are no longer bent at the waist, and simultaneously push up onto the left elbow and forearm and straighten your legs so that your entire torso and your thigh are off the mat. Your body should form a straight line from you right shoulder down to your right ankle (see picture 2).
6. Hold this position while abdominal bracing for 10 seconds.
7. Bend your knees and hips together and slowly lower yourself onto the mat in the start position.
8. Rest for five seconds, then repeat steps 4–8. Perform two sets of four reps on each side. Rest for 60 seconds between sets.
9. Swap to the right side of your body and repeat steps 1–8 on the other side.

MODIFIED SIDE BRIDGE
If you are not yet able to perform this exercise, you can use a modified version in the interim:

Cross your arms over your chest. Perform abdominal bracing. Slowly raise your head up so it is in line with your spine, straighten your legs and raise both feet 6–8 cm off the ground while keeping them together. Continue to hold your body in a straight line (see pictures 3 and 4). You can use the same number of reps and sets as above.

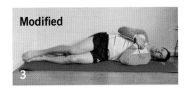

Standard

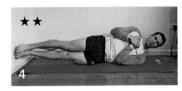

★ ★ ★

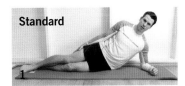

Modified

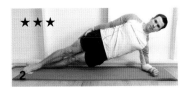

★ ★

TIPS: Try to keep your torso rigid and in a straight line, and don't allow your pelvis to drop down. Avoid letting your knees separate. Swap sides every two sets to allow each side to rest.

Primary muscles worked: Internal and external obliques, transversus abdominis and the quadratus lumborum.

CAUTIONS: Avoid these exercises if you are unable to bear weight on your elbows or forearms, shoulders or lateral thighs.

Side bridge: advanced and expert

ADVANCED

1. Begin by lying in the start position for the standard side bridge exercise.
2. Place your left hand under the shoulder or just to the side in a comfortable position.
3. Perform abdominal bracing.
4. Push your hips forward until you are no longer bent at the waist, and simultaneously push up onto your left elbow and forearm so that your entire torso and thigh are off the mat (see picture 1). You should form a straight line from your shoulder down to your ankle.
5. From this position slowly rotate your right shoulder and hip forward in unison, as though you are reaching underneath yourself. Then rotate back to the start position.
6. Repeat this twist four to six times.
7. Bend your knees and hips, and slowly lower yourself back down onto the mat.
8. Rest for 30 seconds, then repeat steps 3–6 on the same side for four reps.
9. Perform two sets of four reps on each side. Rest for 60 seconds between sets.

EXPERT

1. For Expert level, lie face-down with your knees and feet together.
2. Place both elbows at your sides, keeping both forearms and hands flat on the mat and parallel to your body.
3. Perform abdominal bracing.
4. Rise up to a front plank position (see picture 3).
5. From this position, slowly rotate your right shoulder and torso backward in unison until you reach the side plank position (see picture 4).
6. Pause for one second, then slowly rotate your right shoulder and hip forward (in unison) until you are again in a front plank position.
7. Now, slowly rotate your left shoulder and torso backward (in unison) until you have again reached the side plank position (see picture 5).
8. Repeat steps 4–7 for two sets of four reps. Rest for 30 seconds between reps and 60 seconds between sets.

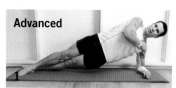

Advanced

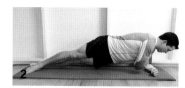

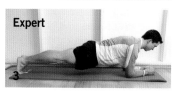

Expert

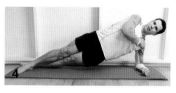

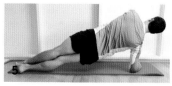

TIPS: Keep your torso rigid and your body in a straight line. Be sure to rotate your entire body in one motion and keep your neck in line with the rest of your spine. Swap sides every two sets to allow each side to rest.

Primary muscles worked: Internal and external obliques, transversus abdominis and quadratus lumborum.

CAUTIONS: Avoid this exercise if you are unable to twist your torso or bear weight on your wrists, elbows or forearms, shoulders or the sides of your feet.

Front plank: remedial and half front plank

REMEDIAL

1. Begin by facing a sturdy wall and standing approximately 50 cm to 1 m away from it, depending on your height, with your feet shoulder-width apart.
2. Perform abdominal bracing.
3. Lean forward until you can place both forearms on the wall in a horizontal position, at shoulder height. Maintain a rigid torso and keep your body in a straight line
4. Hold this position while abdominal bracing for 10 seconds.

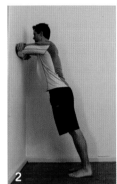
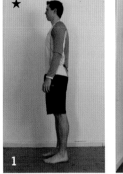

5. Keeping rigid through the body, slowly push yourself back to an upright standing position by straightening your arms and pushing off the wall.
6. Rest for 60 seconds, then repeat for a total of four reps.

HALF FRONT PLANK

If you find the remedial exercise above too easy, use the half front plank instead.

1. Lie face-down on an exercise mat with your knees and feet together and the knees bent to about 90 degrees (see picture 3).
2. Place both elbows at your sides, keeping both forearms and hands flat on the mat and parallel to your body.
3. Perform abdominal bracing.
4. Push up onto your elbows and knees while maintaining a straight spine. You should have a straight line all the way from your shoulders down to your knees (see picture 4).
5. Hold this position while abdominal bracing for 10 seconds.
6. Slowly lower yourself back to the start position by bending your elbows as though you are lowering yourself after a push-up.
7. Rest for five seconds, then repeat steps 3–6. Perform two sets of four reps. Rest for 60 seconds between sets.

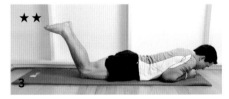
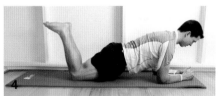

TIPS: Keep your torso rigid and in a straight line. For the remedial front plank, only perform this exercise on a non-slip wall.

Primary muscles worked: Internal and external obliques, rectus abdominis, transversus abdominis and the quadratus lumborum.

CAUTIONS: Avoid this exercise is you are unable to bear weight on your knees, shoulders, elbows, wrists or hands. Be careful not to extend your spine (bend it backwards).

Front plank

1. Lie face-down on an exercise mat. Place your elbows next to your body and keep both forearms flat on the mat. Place your knees and feet together (see picture 1).
2. Perform abdominal bracing.
3. Push up onto your elbows and toes while maintaining a straight spine. You should have a straight line all the way from your shoulders down to your heels (see picture 2).
4. Hold this position while abdominal bracing for 10 seconds.
5. Slowly lower yourself back to the start position. Rest for five seconds, then repeat. Perform a total of two sets of four reps, resting for 60 seconds between sets.

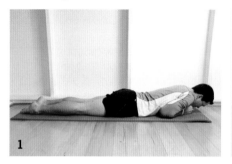
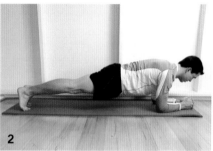

TIPS: Do not arch or bend your low back. Try to maintain a straight spine. You may begin to shake a little near the end of the hold time as you fatigue; this is normal, and it should decrease with a few weeks of consistent training.

Primary muscles worked: Rectus abdominis, transversus abdominis, external and internal obliques.

CAUTIONS: Avoid this exercise if you are unable to bear weight on your elbows, forearms, shoulders or toes.

Front plank: pulsed and advanced

1. Lie face-down on an exercise mat. Place both elbows next to your body and keep your forearms flat on the mat. Place your knees and feet together.
2. Perform abdominal bracing.
3. Push up onto your elbows and toes while maintaining a neutral spine. You should have a straight line all the way from your shoulders down to your heels.

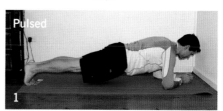

PULSED

4. Push your body forward by pointing your toes, shifting your torso forward over your elbows, then push backward to your original position.
5. Repeat step 4 in quick pulse-like successions.
6. Perform 10 pulses, then lower yourself down onto the mat and rest for five seconds.
7. Repeat steps 4–6 for two sets of four reps. Rest for 60 seconds between sets.

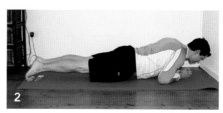

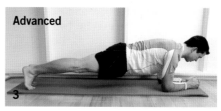

ADVANCED

4. Slowly lift your right elbow 2 cm off the mat for two seconds, then lower it back onto the mat (see picture 4).
5. Raise your left elbow off the mat for two seconds, then lower it back onto the mat (see picture 5).
6. Repeat steps 4–5 for two sets of 10 reps. Rest for 60 seconds between sets.

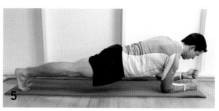

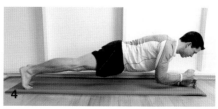

TIPS: Only increase the bend of your elbows when shifting forward for a pulse. Avoid raising your bottom higher than your shoulders. Avoid shifting your hips and pelvis from side to side while raising the elbows off the mat. Maintain a neutral spine throughout the exercise and avoid allowing your chest or pelvis to sag down towards the mat.

Primary muscles worked: Rectus abdominis, transversus abdominis, external and internal obliques.

CAUTIONS: Avoid this exercise if you are unable to bear weight on your elbows or forearms, shoulders or toes.

Front plank with arm and leg lift

1. Lie face-down on an exercise mat. Position your elbows at your sides and keep both forearms flat on the mat. Place your knees and feet together (see picture 1).
2. Perform abdominal bracing.
3. Push up onto your elbows and toes while maintaining a neutral spine (see picture 2).
4. Slowly lift your left elbow and right foot approximately 5 cm off the mat for two seconds (see picture 3), then return them to the mat.
5. Lift your right elbow and left foot off the mat for two seconds (see picture 4), then return them to the mat.
6. Perform two sets of 10 reps, swapping sides for each rep. Rest for 60 seconds between sets.

TIPS: Avoid shifting your hips and pelvis from side to side while raising your elbow and foot off the mat. Avoid raising your leg higher than the level of your bottom. Avoid raising your shoulder above your ear, as this can cause twisting in the spine.

Primary muscles worked: Rectus abdominis, transversus abdominis, external and internal obliques, hamstrings, gluteus maximus and erector spinae.

CAUTIONS: Avoid this exercise if you are unable to bear weight on your elbows or forearms, shoulders or toes.

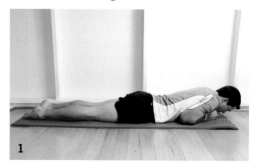

1

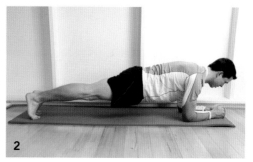

2

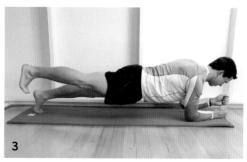

3

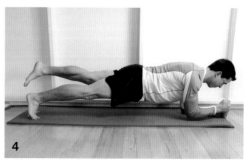

4

Front plank with side tap outs

1. Lie face-down on an exercise mat. Position your elbows at your sides and keep both forearms flat on the mat. Place your knees and feet together.
2. Perform abdominal bracing.
3. Push up onto your elbows and toes until you achieve the front plank position.

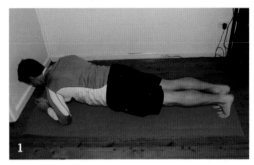

4. Slowly lift your right foot off the mat and move your leg away from your body as far as you can, and gently tap the floor with your toes, without bearing weight (see picture 2).
5. Return your right foot to the starting position.
6. Repeat step 4 with your left foot (see picture 4).
7. Return your left foot to the starting position.

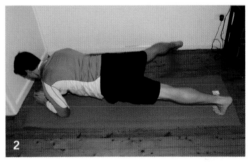

8. Perform two sets of 10 tap outs, swapping sides for each tap out. Rest for 60 seconds between sets.

TIPS: Avoid shifting your hips and pelvis from side to side while raising your foot off the mat. Avoid raising your bottom during the exercise.

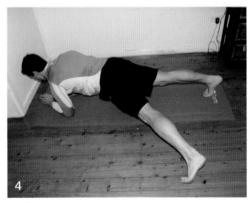

Primary muscles worked: Rectus abdominis, transversus abdominis, external and internal obliques, hamstrings, gluteus max/med/minimus, tensor fasciae latae and erector spinae.

CAUTIONS: Avoid this exercise if you are unable to bear weight on your elbows or forearms, shoulders or toes.

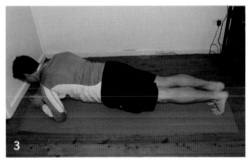

Curl-up: beginner and intermediate

BEGINNER

1. Begin flat on your back with the right knee bent so that your foot is flat on the floor and close to your body.
2. Place your hands under the small of your back (just above your pelvis), one hand on top of the other.
3. Perform abdominal bracing.
4. Keeping elbows in contact with the mat, slowly raise your head, neck and shoulders a few centimetres off the mat so the tips of your shoulder blades are just touching the mat.
5. Hold this position while abdominal bracing for 10 seconds (see picture 1).
6. Slowly lower your head and shoulders back to the start position.
7. Rest for five seconds, then repeat steps 3–6.
8. Perform two sets of 4–6 reps. Rest for 60 seconds between sets.
9. Once you have completed all the sets and reps with the right leg bent, do the next set of exercises with the left leg bent.

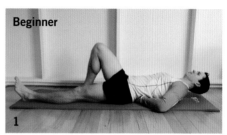

Beginner
1

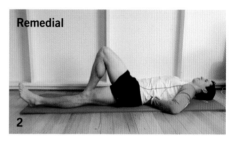

Remedial
2

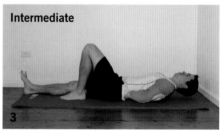

Intermediate
3

REMEDIAL

If the beginner curl-up proves too difficult or places too much strain on your neck, you can decrease the difficulty of the exercise. Simply change step 4 to: Slowly lift your head so that it almost leaves the mat. There should be no gap between your head and the mat (see picture 2). Follow steps 5–10 as described above.

INTERMEDIATE

The Intermediate version of this exercise is more challenging. It is performed in the same manner with the addition of raising both elbows just off the mat after step 3 (see picture 3).

TIPS: Avoid tucking in or poking out your chin. Focus on bending through the mid back. Pushing your tongue to the top of your mouth, just behind the front teeth, will contract your deep neck flexors. Be sure not to hold your breath. To increase the difficulty of this exercise you can cross your arms and grasp your opposite shoulder instead.

Primary muscles worked: Rectus abdominis, obliques and transversus abdominis.

Curl-up: advanced and expert

ADVANCED

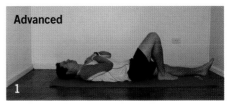

Advanced

1. Begin flat on your back with the right knee bent so that your foot is flat on the floor and close to your body.
2. Lightly place the fingertips of both hands on your forehead with your elbows bent outwards.
3. Perform abdominal bracing.
4. Slowly raise your head, neck and shoulders off the mat so the tips of your shoulder blades are just touching the mat; keep your neck straight.
5. Extend both arms over your head while clasping your hands together (see picture 3).
6. Hold this position while abdominal bracing for 10 seconds.
7. Slowly lower your arms, head and shoulders back to the start position.
8. Rest for five seconds, then repeat steps 3–7.
9. Perform two sets of 4–6 reps. Rest for 60 seconds between sets.
10. Once you have completed all the sets and reps with the right leg bent, do the next set of exercises with the left leg bent.

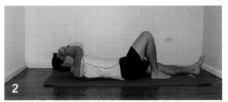

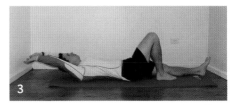

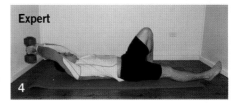

Expert

EXPERT

For a more challenging version of this exercise, modify step 5 as follows: Have a small dumbbell ready above your head, positioned vertically so you can grab it when you extend your arms over your head. Extend both arms over your head and grab the dumbbell off the floor with both hands, and raise it a few centimetres off the ground. Perform step 6 as above. Then carefully lower the dumbbell back to the floor. Perform the same number of reps and sets as above.

TIPS: Avoid tucking in or poking out your chin. Focus on bending through the mid back. Pushing your tongue to the top of your mouth, just behind the front teeth, will contract your deep neck flexors. If performing the expert version of the exercise, start with a small weight (1–2 kg) before progressing to heavier weights. If you are unable to fully extend both arms over your head, try only raising one arm, or keep your elbows flexed so your hands aren't extended too far over your head.

Primary muscles worked: Rectus abdominis, obliques and transversus abdominis.

CAUTIONS: Do not perform this exercise if you have neck instability or if it aggravates your neck pain. Be careful when replacing the dumbbell on the floor so you don't knock it over or place it on an uneven surface.

Bird dog: remedial (arms or legs only)

1. Begin on your hands and knees, with both hands placed directly beneath your shoulders and both knees directly beneath your hips.
2. Place your spine in a neutral position. To find neutral, fully flex your spine down towards the floor, then fully extend the spine up (within a pain-free range). Neutral is found at the mid-point between both extremes.
3. Perform abdominal bracing.
4. Slowly raise your right hand or your right knee (depending on whether you are performing arms or legs) approximately 5 cm off the mat. Keep the rest of the body still and maintain the neutral spine position.
5. Hold this position while abdominal bracing for 10 seconds.
6. Slowly lower your raised arm or leg back to the start position, then raise your left arm or leg.
7. Perform two sets of four reps for each arm or leg. Rest for 60 seconds between sets.

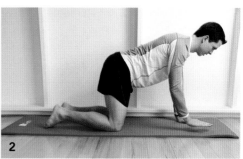

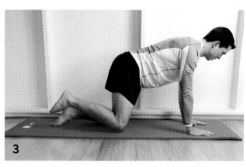

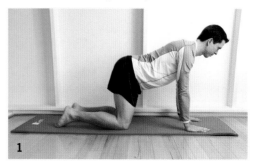

TIPS: Avoid over-extending the arms or legs. Stay rigid through the low back and pelvis, while keeping a neutral spine.

Primary muscles worked: Gluteus maximus, hamstrings, transversus abdominis, lumbar multifidus, longissimus, iliocostalis thoracis and lumborum.

CAUTIONS: Avoid this exercise if you are unable to bear weight through your arms, hands or wrists, or your knees. Be careful not to flex or extend your spine into a painful range when finding your neutral spine position.

Bird dog: beginner

1. Begin on your hands and knees, with both hands placed directly beneath your shoulders and both knees directly beneath your hips (see picture 1).
2. Place your spine in a neutral position. To find neutral, fully flex your spine down towards the floor, then fully extend the spine up (within a pain-free range). Neutral is found at the mid-point between both extremes.
3. Perform abdominal bracing.
4. Slowly lift your left arm and at the same time extend your right leg while keeping your right foot in contact with the floor.
5. Raise your arm to as close to shoulder height as is comfortable. Keep the rest of your body still and maintain a neutral spine position.
6. Hold this position while abdominal bracing for two seconds (see picture 2).
7. Slowly and simultaneously return your arm and leg to the start position (see picture 1).
8. Repeat steps 3–7 using your right arm and left leg.
9. Perform two sets of 10 reps. Rest for 60 seconds between sets.

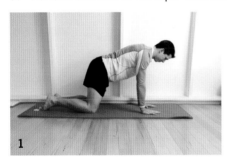
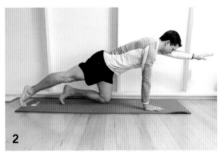

Alternative version: For greater endurance training, this exercise can be done by performing all the repetitions of a set with the right arm and left leg before changing to the opposite arm and leg on the following set.

TIPS: Stay rigid in the low back and pelvis throughout the exercise while maintaining a neutral spine. Avoid raising your hand above the level of your ear, as this can cause twisting in the spine.

Primary muscles worked: Gluteus maximus, hamstrings, transversus abdominis, lumbar multifidus, longissimus, iliocostalis thoracis and lumborum.

CAUTIONS: Avoid this exercise if you are unable to bear weight on your arms or your knees. Be careful not to bend your spine into a painful range when finding your neutral spine position.

Bird dog: intermediate

1. Begin on your hands and knees, with both hands placed directly beneath your shoulders and both knees directly beneath your hips (see picture 1).
2. Place your spine in a neutral position. To find neutral, fully flex your spine down towards the floor, then fully extend the spine up (within a pain-free range). Neutral is found at the mid-point between both extremes.
3. Perform abdominal bracing.
4. Slowly raise your left arm and your right leg at the same time until you reach a comfortable height (see picture 2). Keep the rest of the body still and maintain a neutral spine.
5. Hold this position while abdominal bracing for one second.
6. Slowly and simultaneously lower your arm and leg back down to the start position
7. Without taking a rest, perform steps 3–6 with your right arm and left leg.
8. Perform two sets of 10 reps. Rest for 60 seconds between sets.

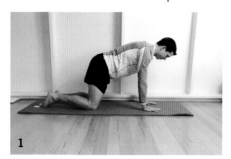 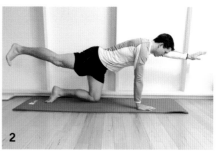

Alternative version: After you become proficient at this exercise, an alternative version can be done by changing step 5 to a 10-second hold, then performing two sets of four reps. Change to the opposite arm and leg for each repetition.

TIPS: Avoid rotating your hip (known as 'hip hiking') and over-extending your arms or legs. Stay rigid in the low back and pelvis throughout the exercise while maintaining a neutral spine. Avoid raising your foot above the level of the buttock. Avoid raising your hand above the level of your ear, as this can cause twisting in the spine.

Primary muscles worked: Gluteus maximus, hamstrings, transversus abdominis, lumbar multifidus, longissimus, iliocostalis thoracis and lumborum.

CAUTIONS: Avoid this exercise if you are unable to bear weight through your upper limbs or your knees. Be careful not to flex or extend your spine into a painful range when finding your neutral spine position.

Bird dog: advanced

1. Begin on your hands and knees, with both hands placed directly beneath your shoulders and both knees directly beneath your hips.
2. Place your spine in a neutral position. To find neutral, fully flex your spine down towards the floor, then fully extend the spine up (within a pain-free range). Neutral is found at the mid-point between both extremes.
3. Perform abdominal bracing.
4. Slowly lift your left arm and fully extend your right leg at the same time until you reach a comfortable height. Keep the rest of your body still and maintain a neutral spine (see picture 1).
5. Slowly lower your arm and leg back to the start position, sweeping the mat with the knee and back of the hand (see picture 2).
6. Repeat steps 3–5 for two sets of five reps on each side. Rest for 60 seconds between sets.

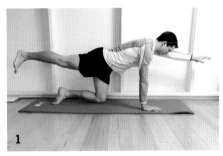

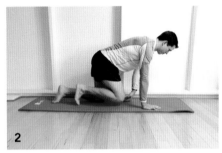

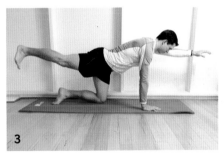

Alternate version: This exercise can easily be made more difficult by adding small wrist and ankle weights.

TIPS: Avoid rotating your hip (known as 'hip hiking'), and over-extending the arms or legs. Stay rigid in the low back and pelvis throughout the exercise, while maintaining a neutral spine.

Primary muscles worked: Gluteus maximus, hamstrings, transversus abdominis, lumbar multifidus, longissimus, iliocostalis thoracis and lumborum.

CAUTIONS: Avoid this exercise if you are unable to bear weight on your arms or knees. Be careful not to bend your spine into a painful range when finding your neutral spine position.

Bird dog: expert

1. Begin on your hands and knees, with both hands placed directly beneath your shoulders and both knees directly beneath your hips.
2. Place your spine in a neutral position. To find neutral, fully flex your spine down towards the floor, then fully extend the spine up (within a pain-free range). Neutral is found at the mid-point between both extremes.
3. Perform abdominal bracing.
4. Draw a square in the air in front of you. Begin by raising your arm and leg so they end up in line with the spine, no higher than the shoulders (see picture 2).
5. Slowly move both limbs approximately 15–30 cm away from your body (see picture 3).
6. Then slowly lower both limbs so that they end up almost touching the floor (see picture 4).
7. Finally, bring both limbs back towards the body to complete the square (see picture 5).
8. Perform two sets of five reps each side. Rest for 60 seconds between sets.

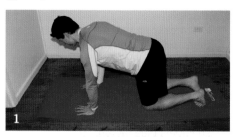

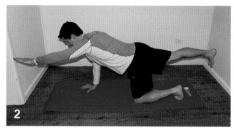

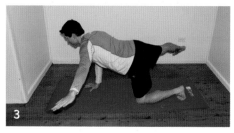

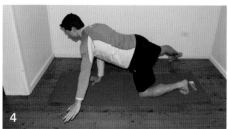

Alternate version: This exercise can easily be made more difficult by adding small wrist and ankle weights.

TIPS: The idea is to draw simultaneous squares with your opposing arm and leg. Avoid shifting your hips to the side while raising the elbow and foot off the mat.

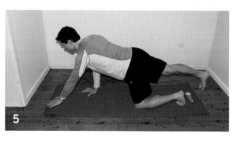

Primary muscles worked: Rectus abdominis, transversus abdominis, external and internal obliques, hamstrings, gluteus maximus and erector spinae.

CAUTIONS: Avoid this exercise if you are unable to bear weight on your arms or knees. Be careful not to flex or extend your spine into a painful range when finding your neutral spine position.

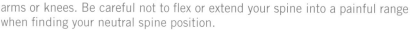

Bridge

BEGINNER

1. Begin by lying flat on your back on an exercise mat with your knees bent so that your feet are flat on the floor at a comfortable position. Both your knees and feet should be about hip-width apart.
2. Place your forearms across your chest and perform abdominal bracing (see picture 1).
3. Slowly raise your bottom off the floor by firmly clenching your buttocks until you reach a height where you form a straight line from your knees to your shoulders (see picture 2).
4. Hold this position for 10 seconds, then slowly lower yourself back into the starting position.
5. Repeat steps 2–4. Perform two sets of four reps. Rest for 60 seconds between sets.

REMEDIAL

If you are not yet able to perform this exercise, use this easier version.

1. Instead of crossing your arms across your chest, place your hands approximately 10 cm away from your body with your palms flat on the floor. Perform abdominal bracing (see picture 3).
2. Slowly raise your bottom off the floor by firmly clenching your buttocks and simultaneously pressing downward with both arms to help raise your pelvis up to a height where you form a straight line from your knees to your shoulders.

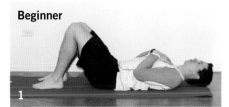

Beginner

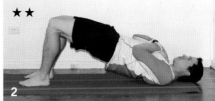

★ ★

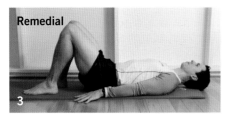

Remedial

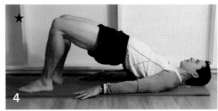

★

TIPS: This is a great exercise for working your hip extensors. Make sure your hips don't begin to sag towards the floor before the time is finished. Using your arms in the remedial version of this exercise will help you lift up your pelvis and maintain balance.

Primary muscles worked: Gluteus maximus, medius and minimus, hamstrings, transversus abdominis, rectus abdominis, and internal and external obliques.

CAUTIONS: Avoid this exercise if you are unable to bear weight on your feet, ankles, knees or upper back. Immediately stop the exercise if you experience any pain greater than mild discomfort.

Bridge: intermediate

1. Begin by lying flat on your back on an exercise mat with your knees bent so that your feet are flat on the floor at a comfortable angle. Both your knees and feet should be about hip-width apart.
2. Place your hands approximately 10 cm away from your body with your palms flat on the floor.
3. Perform abdominal bracing.
4. Slowly raise your bottom off the mat by firmly clenching your buttocks until you reach a height where there is a straight line from knees to your shoulders.
5. Begin to straighten your right leg until it is fully extended and your thighs are parallel (see picture 2). Hold for 10 seconds.
6. Carefully return your foot to the mat and lower yourself back into the starting position. Rest for five seconds.
7. Repeat steps 3–6 with the same leg. Perform two sets of four reps with each leg. Rest for 60 seconds between sets.

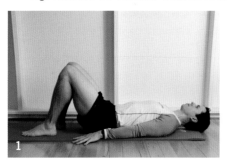 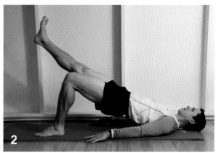

Alternative version: After you become proficient at this exercise, an alternative version of this has you change step 5 so you hold your leg up for only one second, replace the foot on the mat then repeat step 5 with the other leg. Perform two sets of 10 reps.

TIPS: This is a great exercise for working your hip extensors. Make sure your hips don't begin to sag towards the floor before the time is finished.

Primary muscles worked: Gluteus maximus, medius and minimus, hamstrings, transversus abdominis, rectus abdominis, and internal and external obliques.

CAUTIONS: Avoid this exercise if you are unable to bear weight on your feet, ankles, knees or upper back. Immediately stop the exercise if you experience any pain greater than mild discomfort.

Bridge: advanced and expert

ADVANCED

1. Begin by lying flat on your back on an exercise mat with your knees bent so that your feet are flat on the floor at a comfortable angle. Both your knees and feet should be about hip-width apart.
2. Place your arms across your chest and perform abdominal bracing.
3. Slowly raise your bottom off the mat by firmly clenching your buttocks until you reach a height where there is a straight line from your knees to your shoulders.
4. Begin to straighten your right leg until it is fully extended and your thighs are parallel. Hold for one second.
5. Return your foot to the mat and, without lowering your bottom, straighten your left leg until it is fully extended and your thighs are parallel. Hold for one second.
6. Perform two sets of 10 reps. After your final repetition in each set, return your left foot to the mat then slowly lower yourself back into the starting position. Rest for 60 seconds between sets.

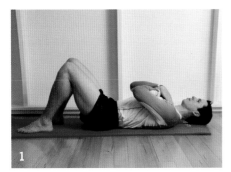 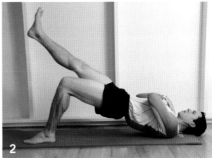

Expert version: At step 4, instead of simply holding your leg extended, you can draw circles (clockwise and counter-clockwise) of varying sizes for 10 seconds. Lower yourself back onto the mat and rest for 5 seconds. Then repeat with opposite leg. Perform two sets of two reps for each leg. Rest for 60 seconds between sets.

TIPS: This is a great exercise for working your hip muscles. Make sure your hips don't begin to sag towards the floor before the time is finished.

Primary muscles worked: Gluteus maximus, medius and minimus, hamstrings, transversus abdominis, rectus abdominis, and internal and external obliques.

CAUTIONS: Avoid this exercise if you are unable to bear weight on your feet, ankles, knees or upper back. Immediately stop the exercise if you experience any pain greater than mild discomfort.

Cat/camel: prone and seated

PRONE

1. Begin on your hands and knees, both hands placed directly beneath your shoulders and both knees beneath your hips. Place your spine in a neutral position.
2. Slowly arch your spine downwards as much as you comfortably can, extend your neck and look up to the ceiling, and stick your bum out (see picture 1). Hold this end position for two seconds.
3. Slowly reverse the movement by rounding your spine (pushing the spine up towards the ceiling), tucking your chin in to your chest, and tucking in your bum (see picture 2). Hold for two seconds.

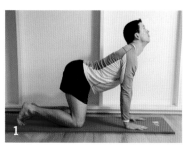

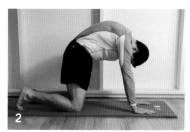

SEATED

1. Sit near the front edge of a chair with your knees hip-width apart, and your feet flat on the ground directly beneath your knees.
2. Curl forward by rounding your spine, tucking your chin and extending your arms forward. Bring your hands together as though you are going to dive into a pool (see picture 3). Hold for two seconds.
3. Slowly reverse the movement by arching your spine as much as you comfortably can, extending your neck and looking up to the ceiling, and pulling your elbows back as if you were trying to bring them together behind your back (see picture 4). Hold for two seconds.
4. Repeat in either position for eight reps (one rep in this case is going both forward and backward).
5. Perform two sets of eight reps. Rest for 60 seconds between sets.

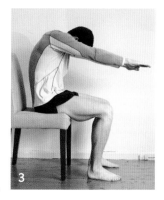

TIPS: This is a mobilisation, not a stretch. Only move to approximately 90 per cent of your maximum range. This exercise helps decrease spinal stiffness and lubricate the joints of the spine. This can be done several times a day and is great for desk workers. Only move within your pain-free range of motion, which range may only be small in the beginning but usually increases if the mobilisation is performed regularly.

Areas being worked: Cervical, thoracic and lumbar vertebrae, abdominals and erector spinae muscles.

CAUTIONS: Avoid the prone version if you are unable to bear weight on your knees, shoulders, elbows and wrists. Immediately stop the exercise if you experience any pain greater than mild discomfort.

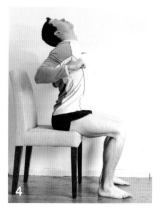

Brügger

1. Begin in a standing position with both arms down at your sides, elbows bent to 90 degrees and both palms facing each other. Take a deep breath.
2. Spread your fingers wide, without straining them.
3. While keeping your thumbs pointed to the ceiling, bend your wrists so your fingers are pointing towards the floor.
4. Now turn your palms upward so they are facing the ceiling (supinate).
5. Keeping your elbows touching your sides, rotate both arms outward as in picture 3.
6. Slowly breathe out as much as you can while depressing your shoulder blades and bringing them close together.
7. Hold this position for as long as it takes you to completely breathe out, then return to the start position.
8. Perform two sets of three reps. Rest for 30 seconds between sets.

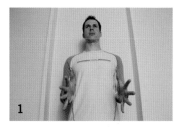

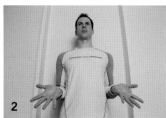

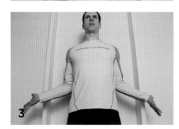

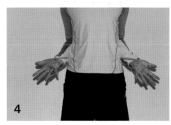

Alternative version: seated
This mobilisation can be performed in a seated position.

Advanced version: Brügger with resistance
A more challenging version of this exercise can also be performed using resistive elastic band. Use a piece about 1.5 m long. Begin by placing the band across your lower back while loosely grasping the ends of the band between your thumbs and index fingers of both hands. Turn your palms so they are in front of you facing away from your body with the elastic in front of your palm and the loose ends hanging in front of the palms. While grasping the band, turn your palms inward so they now face you. Now wrap the band around your hand by reaching over the top of the band with your fingers pointing towards you and then dive under it so the band wraps around the back of your hand but in front of your thumb. Perform the exercise as outlined above from steps 1–5. The final part of the movement involves slowly extending your arms until they are fully extended. Hold this position for one second, then slowly allow the elbows to bend until they are touching the sides of your body (this should take five seconds). Return your hands to the starting position and then repeat the entire movement. Perform two sets of 10 reps once per day.

Primary muscles worked: Middle and lower trapezius, rhomboids and latissimus dorsi.

CAUTIONS: If any symptoms intensify while performing this exercise, stop immediately and consult your practitioner.

Prone lying: sphinx and cobra

These exercises can be done on any surface, but we recommend using either carpet or an exercise mat.

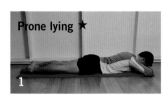
Prone lying ★

PRONE LYING

1. Begin by lying flat on your stomach with your legs fully extended and close together. (Place a pillow under your abdomen if you feel excessive back strain.)
2. Position your arms so that you can overlap your hands and place them under your forehead.
3. Once you have attained this position, hold it for 60 seconds. This exercise can be performed for 1–5 minutes up to once every hour.
4. Progress this mobilisation by placing one or two closed fists under your chin (see picture 2).

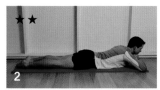
★★

SPHINX

1. Place your elbows shoulder-width apart and keep both forearms flat on the mat, next to your body, with your hands below your throat.
2. Clasp your hands together and rest your chin on your hands.

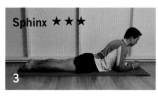
Sphinx ★★★

3. While keeping your pelvis on the mat, slowly extend your spine by rising up onto your forearms.
4. Continue to extend your back until you either feel a good stretch in your back or experience some low back discomfort, then stop.
5. Once you have extended into a position you can comfortably maintain, hold that position for 10 seconds.

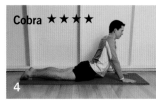
Cobra ★★★★

6. Gently lower yourself back down to the start position and immediately rise up again and hold for 10 seconds.
7. Perform 10 reps with a 10 second hold up to four times per day.

COBRA

1. Place both hands on the mat as if you were going to perform a push-up.
2. While keeping your pelvis and legs on the mat, slowly extend your spine by fully straightening out your elbows.
3. Once you have extended into a position you can comfortably maintain, hold that position for 10 seconds.
4. Gently lower yourself back down to the start position and immediately push up again, and hold for 10 seconds.
5. Perform 10 reps with a 10 second hold up to 4 times per day.

TIPS: These exercises were designed for patients with disc herniations and sciatica. The goal is to get your pain to centralise—the pain will decrease in the lower limbs but may temporarily increase in the low back.

CAUTIONS: It is normal to experience some discomfort in the low back while performing the exercise, but not in your legs. If leg pain intensifies during or after the exercise, do not perform the exercise again until you can consult with your practitioner. Those with spinal stenosis or severe facet joint arthrosis should avoid this exercise.

Split stance

The split stance is simply a standing posture where one foot is placed slightly ahead of the other in a balanced and stable position. The split stance is helpful in many ways. It allows for easier weight transference backwards and forwards, and it allows you to reach higher or farther with one arm than possible in a straight stance. The split stance significantly reduces unwanted strain on the neck and low back by promoting a more neutral posture at the pelvis. Since you can shift your weight backwards and forwards, it is easier to bring items closer to your centre of gravity, thereby reducing load on your spine.

When you reach forward to lift an object you place greater strain on your spine when standing with your feet side by side than with the split stance. This is because when lifting, the farther an object is from your centre of gravity, the greater the lever arm is. A lever arm is the distance a load is from the centre of gravity (fulcrum) of a lever. As a lever arm gets longer, the relative load of the object being lifted increases. For example, if you were to grab a 5-kg weight and hold it by your side, and then hold the weight at arm's length in front of you, you would notice that the weight feels a lot heavier when held out at arm's length. By adopting a split stance you shorten the lever arm, which effectively reduces the effect of the weight you are lifting and places less load on the spine.

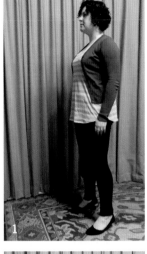

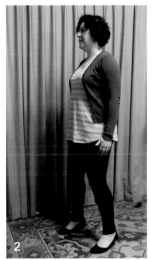

1. Begin in a standing position with your feet approximately hip-width apart.
2. Place one foot approximately half a foot length forward of the other and shift your centre of gravity forward so your body is centred (equidistant) over your two feet.
3. From this position, bend the knees just a bit so they are not in a locked position.

TIPS: It shouldn't matter which foot goes in front of the other, but most people have a predilection for placing a certain foot in front.

Rolling over and getting out of bed

Rolling over in bed can be very painful for people with a back problem. It's also almost unavoidable due to the fact that most of us change position approximately 13 times over eight hours of sleep. In this example, we are going to show you how to roll from your back to your left side and get out of bed from the left side of the bed.

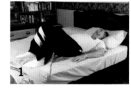

1. Before you start to move your spine, make sure that you are free of your bed sheets so that you will not be inhibited when you move.
2. Bend both knees so that your feet are flat on the bed.
3. Perform abdominal bracing.

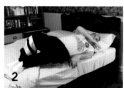

4. Continue to hold the abdominal bracing while carefully using your legs to lift your bottom a few centimetres off the bed and shift it a few centimetres to the right.
5. At the same time, raise your right shoulder off the bed and begin rotating your entire body as one unit to the left. Relax. You have now successfully rolled to one side.

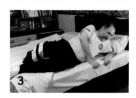

6. From this position, shift your body to the edge of the bed.
7. Perform abdominal bracing again.
8. Slowly drop both legs off the side of the bed and use your left elbow and right hand to push yourself up into a sitting position.

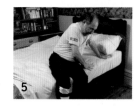

9. Slide your bottom to the edge of the bed so that you are almost falling off the edge and place your hands palms-down on the mattress beside your thighs.
10. Place both your feet hip-width apart on the floor in a split stance position (the strongest leg nearest the bed and the other leg a few centimetres ahead of it).

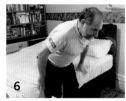

11. Perform abdominal bracing.
12. Extend both arms to push off the mattress and simultaneously push up with your legs until you achieve a standing position.
13. It may be difficult to stand perfectly upright immediately, so give yourself a moment to get used to standing. You can either stand in the same position for a minute or walk around until you are more comfortable.

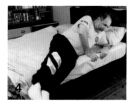

TIPS: If you are getting up in the middle of the night, we suggest turning on a light to avoid tripping. This will also mean that if your back spasms you can grab onto something for support. If your back spasms while you are trying to roll over, stop moving and wait for the spasm to subside before attempting to move again.

CAUTIONS: Taking sleeping pills can be problematic because they cause you to pass out, which turns off your body's pain-protection mechanisms.

Getting up from a seated position

Most people with healthy backs take the simple act of getting up from a seated position for granted. For those suffering with acute or chronic back pain, this act can be difficult if not impossible without assistance. There are, however, a few tricks available that can facilitate the act of moving from a seated to a standing position while making the movement safer, less painful and easier to perform. For this example, we demonstrate how to get up from a chair; however, the basic principles can be applied to getting up from most seated positions. To get into a seated position, follow the same procedure in reverse.

1. Begin by sliding your bottom forward on the chair so you end up near the front edge with your knees hip-width apart. Your legs should be bent to approximately 90 degrees and your feet should be flat on the ground.
2. Place the foot of your stronger leg slightly behind the front edge of the chair, and the other foot positioned so that your heel is directly under your knee.
3. Place both hands palms-down on the base or armrests.
4. Perform abdominal bracing.
5. Extend both arms to push off and simultaneously push up with your legs until you achieve a standing position.
6. It may be difficult to stand perfectly upright right away, so give your back a minute to get used to standing. You can either stand in the same position for a moment or walk around a bit to loosen your back.

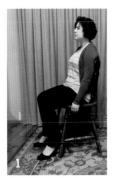 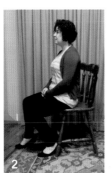 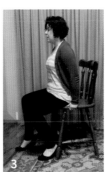 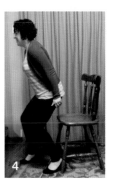

TIPS: The abdominal bracing will help stabilise your spine when you begin to move and can often avoid unnecessary pain during the movement.

CAUTIONS: Be careful that you don't slip off when you move to the edge of the seat. Before going to sit down, always make sure the object you intend to sit on is able to support your weight and will not slip or slide away from you.

Hip hinge

The hip hinge involves flexing at the hips while maintaining a neutral spine. This is done most notably by Olympic weightlifters. It is easier to bend forward using the hip hinge than bending with the low back, because it recruits several powerful muscles. Using the hip hinge can save your back from unnecessary compression over a lifetime, and possibly prevent you from damaging your back.

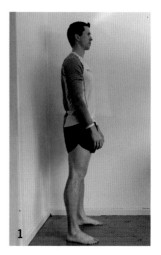

1. Stand facing away from a sturdy wall that can support your entire body weight. Place your feet approximately hip-width apart with your heels about 30 cm away from the wall.
2. Slightly bend both knees and push your bottom backwards while keeping your head and chest up, and your spine in a neutral position.
3. Push your bottom backwards until it is just touching the wall and hold your arms out in front of you.
4. Hold this position for one second—be sure not to lean against the wall.
5. Return to the upright position by thrusting your hips forward and straightening your knees.
6. Perform two sets of 10 reps. Rest for 60 seconds between sets.

Once you get the hang of it, move your feet further away from the wall in 5 cm increments, until you can no longer touch the wall with your bottom. That will be the end range for your hip hinge.

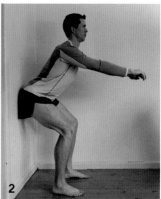

TIPS: This exercise is meant to teach you how to bend properly without compromising your low back. Avoid bending your low back throughout this movement. This exercise can be done with dumbbells if you want to make it more difficult, but weights should only be added if you have mastered the movement and can easily perform three sets of 15 repetitions.

Primary muscles worked: Gluteus maximus, medius and minimus, psoas, hamstrings and quadriceps.

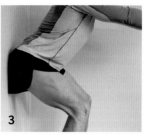

CAUTIONS: Discontinue this exercise if it aggravates your back pain, and consult your practitioner before trying it again. Do not perform this exercise on a slippery surface.

Getting in and out of a car

Prolonged sitting in a car can cause or perpetuate a back problem. While this technique will not necessarily be painless, it should help to reduce the pain the movement can cause.

1. Park in a car space that has enough room for you to fully open your door.
2. Move the seat back as far as it will go, allowing you more room to move.
3. Open the door as wide as possible.
4. Hold onto the top of the steering wheel with your left hand, reach out with the right hand and grab hold of the car roof. Use these as leverage to pivot your body. Place your right foot on the ground.
5. Continue pivoting your body until you can place the left foot on the ground next to the right one.
6. Gently slide your bottom forward to the edge of the seat. Place your right hand on the top of the doorframe while keeping your left hand on the steering wheel.
7. Perform abdominal bracing.
8. Have your feet as far back as possible. Lean out of the car while keeping a neutral spine position. Use your left hand to push yourself up while simultaneously pulling straight down on the doorframe with your right hand.
9. Keep your head up and your knees bent throughout the movement. Use the hip-hinge movement to rise up to a standing position. Do not force your back into a fully upright position if it is not ready—it may take a few minutes for a tight back to straighten up.
10. To get into your car, follow the same procedure in reverse.

This movement strategy may take a little longer than getting out of a car as you're used to; however, you will be able to get in and out with a lot less pain by using it.

TIPS: Abdominal bracing will help stabilise your spine and can help avoid unnecessary pain with this movement.

CAUTIONS: Be careful when grabbing the doorframe if it is wet, as this could cause you to lose your grip and potentially fall. Be careful not to pull the door towards yourself, as this could cause the door to slam into you. Cars that are very low to the ground may prove more difficult to get in and out of; on the other hand, high vehicles can present the problem of falling out of the vehicle onto the ground.

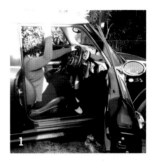

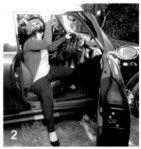

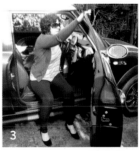

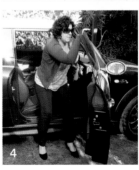

Getting up from a fall

This movement strategy will decrease the risk of causing further injury to yourself when getting up after a fall.

1. Before trying to move, calm and compose yourself.
2. Perform a quick head-to-toe assessment of your body to determine if you are injured, such as any open wounds or broken bones.
3. Make sure that you are free and clear of any objects that may have fallen with you.
4. If you are injured or can't move, do not attempt to get up. Call for help, or wait until you can attract someone's attention to come and help you. Only if you can move and believe you are able to stand should you attempt the following movement strategy.
5. If you have fallen onto your side or back, try to get onto your stomach by performing a log-roll manoeuvre.
6. Once you are on your stomach, position the arm and leg of the strongest side of your body underneath you.
7. Push yourself up onto your hands and knees.
8. Now crawl over to any sturdy support you can reach, such as a chair or bed, to help yourself up.
9. Reach up to the support with both hands. Try to always maintain at least three points of contact to support yourself. Use the chair to support your weight while you position the foot of your strongest leg underneath your knee so you end up in a single-leg kneeling position.
10. Perform abdominal bracing.
11. From this position, push yourself to an upright position.
12. If you feel that you are uninjured and strong enough to walk, you may do so. However, if you are unsure, sit down and re-assess the situation.

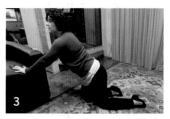
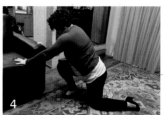
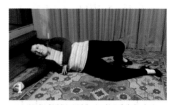
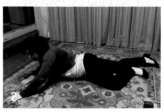
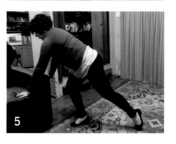

TIPS: Take your time when getting up; if you get halfway through the procedure and need to take a break, that's fine. The task is easier to accomplish when you are not fatigued.

CAUTIONS: Do not get up in this manner if you are unable to bear weight on your knees. This is only one possible way to get up from a fall; it may not be the most appropriate movement strategy for everyone or in every situation.

pads), convection (hydrotherapy, fluidotherapy) or radiation (infrared lamps). Conduction is the transmission of energy from direct contact of a thermal source. Convection is the transmission of energy through movement of fluid or gases resulting in a variation of temperature. Radiation is energy transfer where energetic particles travel through medium or space in the form of electric and magnetic fields that make up electromagnetic waves. Although usually safe, be careful using these strategies as devices can become excessively hot and may cause burns. Microwavable heat bags have been known to explode or spontaneously combust.

Special temperature-sensitive nerve endings called thermoreceptors are activated by changes in skin temperature. Once activated these receptors send nerve signals that block nociception (pain signalling) within the spinal cord. Topical heat, physically applied to the skin, stimulates another type of specialised nerve endings called proprioceptors. Proprioceptors detect physical changes in tissue pressure and movement. As with thermoreceptors, proprioceptors can block the transmission of pain signals to the brain. The activation of these receptors within the spinal cord reduces muscle tone, relaxes painful muscles and enhances tissue blood flow. The therapeutic range for heat packs lies between 40°C and 45°C. Superficial heat elevates the temperature of tissues and provides the greatest effect at 0.5 cm or less from the surface of the skin.

Reasons to have this treatment
Thermotherapy deals with the management of acute and chronic pain, joint stiffness and muscle spasm or guarding.

Reasons this treatment might not be suitable for you
Thermotherapy treatment should not be applied over regions of acute injury, inflammation, bleeding, tumours, impaired sensation and inflamed varicose veins, abdomens of pregnant women or patients with mental impairment. Thermotherapy should never be used over a new or open wound.

Treatment effects
The purported effects include dilated blood vessels, increased metabolic rate, increased **collagen** extensibility, increased nerve conduction, increased pain threshold and decreased muscle tone and spasms.

Positive attributes

Heat is easily available, can be used at home, is relatively inexpensive and safe, and, when effective, can provide immediate and obvious relief. Infrared lamps that use shorter wavelengths are able to penetrate deeper than using other methods. Moist heat has a better heating potential and works faster than dry heat.

Negative attributes

Infrared lamps can be a fire hazard. Skin burns can occur with any form of thermotherapy if proper safety precautions are not followed.

Side effects

Common adverse effects include mild to moderate skin burns. Certain conditions make patients more susceptible to burns, such as diabetes, multiple sclerosis, poor circulation and spinal cord injuries. Whirlpool and other types of hydrotherapy have a risk of infections of the skin, urogenital and pulmonary systems. Heat therapy may exacerbate an inflammatory reaction.

Recommendations

Precautions should be taken when applying heat over areas with impaired circulation, fluid retention, superficial metal implants or open wounds. Do not use heat therapy if you tend to overheat, have cardiac issues or an acute inflammatory disorder, or if you have low blood pressure or are prone to fainting when heating large body areas. If you are being treated for rheumatoid arthritis, heat therapies should be used with caution because increased inflammation may occur.

Proof of effectiveness

Most studies show heat therapy to be a beneficial adjunct. A heat wrap can reduce pain and disability and these effects can last for up to three months. Unfortunately, the relief may not be dramatic.

Electrical muscle stimulation

Muscle stimulation—also referred to as Russian current, neuromuscular electrical stimulation (NMES) or electrical muscle stimulation

(EMS)—is a form of electrotherapy commonly used for the rehabilitation of muscles following injury or stroke. EMS is technically almost identical to a TENS device (see below); however, EMS produces a current that is powerful enough to evoke a muscle contraction. EMS delivers an electrical current through superficial electrodes placed on the skin, causing one or more muscles to contract, which is thought to promote blood supply and help strengthen the affected muscle. By provoking muscle contractions in the area being stimulated, EMS acts as a counterirritant stimulus, reducing muscle spasm, and increasing muscle strength and endurance. The treatment generally lasts from 10 to 30 minutes, and can be applied as often as twice per day (separated by three to four hours).

Reasons to have this treatment
Signs include muscle weakness or disuse atrophy, pain, restriction of joint motion, muscle re-education, oedema, muscle spasm, muscle strains, pain due to muscle spasm, during cast immobilisation.

Reasons this treatment might not be suitable for you
Avoid use over the front neck region, heart, across the chest, areas of impaired sensation, abdomen if pregnant, a pacemaker, implanted defibrillator or any other implanted electrical device or over skin lesions (cuts, abrasions, contusions). Avoid if the patient has venous or arterial thrombosis or thrombophlebitis (inflammation of veins and blood clots).

Treatment effects
This assists muscle hypertrophy (growth), muscle re-education, slows the rate of bone loss, strengthens muscles, maintains or increases range of motion, provides feedback to enhance voluntary muscle control, removes metabolic wastes, mechanically stimulates muscle fibres, increases local blood circulation, and inhibits spasticity and muscle spasm. It can increase body temperature, heart rate and metabolism.

Positive attributes
EMS can be used on immobilised body parts. It promotes an early active range of motion in post-urgical and immobilised limbs. It can prevent complications from immobility such as deep vein thrombosis (DVTs) and osteoporosis.

Negative attributes

Treatment focused on pain may psychologically reinforce a patient's expectation that they won't break the cycle of pain or may indirectly entice patients to take a less active approach to pain management, which may hinder progress towards recovery. The peripheral nerves must be intact for muscle stimulation to work (it won't work if there is nerve damage).

Side effects

A common adverse effect of EMS is minor skin irritations. Skin burns are a rare occurrence and are generally associated with inappropriate use, such as prolonged or continuous use, incorrect placement or settings.

Recommendations

While this therapy may be very useful it is important that you progress to traditional weight training as quickly as possible.

Proof of effectiveness

EMS combined with exercise therapy has been found to be an effective adjunctive treatment for non-acute low back pain. For muscle rehabilitation, a 20 per cent increase in muscle size can be achieved after eight weeks of treatment.

Exercise therapy

This has been used as a treatment therapy for back pain for a very long time. Exercise therapy encompasses a diverse group of interventions that vary in type, intensity, frequency, duration of exercise and the setting in which it is provided. These features make it extremely difficult to accurately assess how well exercise therapy works for various conditions. There is tremendous variation in people's response to exercise; most will achieve moderate improvements, some will achieve quick or significant gains, while others may have only minor improvements. The aim of exercise therapy is to restore normal function and behaviour in patients with low back pain. Exercise therapy is generally provided by four methods:

1. Home exercises only—where you initially meet with a therapist who provides an exercise program with no supervision or follow-up.

2. Supervised home exercises—where you initially meet with a therapist who provides an exercise program and a follow-up session is scheduled at least every six weeks.
3. Group supervision—where you attend supervised exercise-therapy sessions with two or more participants.
4. Individual supervision—where you receive one-on-one supervised exercise therapy sessions.

Reasons to have this treatment

This is suitable for chronic back pain, muscle weakness, lack of muscle endurance, joint hypermobility or instability, poor cardiovascular fitness, poor functional movement, inability to perform activities of daily living, ankylosing spondylitis, osteoarthritis, Parkinson's disease and for patients who have suffered a stroke.

Reasons this treatment might not be suitable for you

There are a number of conditions for which exercise may be counterproductive or even dangerous. If you have one of the following conditions, seek medical advice before starting a therapeutic exercise program: aortic aneurysm or stenosis, heart attack, heart infection, pulmonary embolism, crescendo angina, thrombophlebitis, rapid weak pulse, acute infection. Relative contraindications include heart conditions such as enlargement, untreated hypertension, compensated congestive heart failure, irregular therapy, ventricular ectopic activity, aneurysm; chronic or recurrent infectious diseases; and uncontrolled metabolic disorders (such as diabetes or low thyroid activity). Some conditions may require imposed limitations or special exercise prescription or both. Some patients may require ongoing medical monitoring or an initial supervised session before being approved for exercise therapy.

Treatment effects

Exercise causes the release of endorphins, which are described as the feel good hormone. It also maintains or improves bone density and contributes to muscle growth.

Positive attributes

Exercise therapy can be done by anyone as long as their physical capabilities and condition are taken into account. Exercise therapy can often be done out of the clinic and may not require the use of any equipment. On top of the prescribed exercise's intended purpose, such as increasing strength or endurance, exercise has a positive effect on both the hormonal and metabolic systems of the body.

Negative attributes

Exercise can be difficult and painful for some. It can take several weeks before any significant changes are observed. Some of the improvements gained from the therapy are lost within weeks of stopping exercise therapy.

Side effects

Common side effects include mild to moderate muscle soreness during or after exercise, light-headedness, muscle cramping, hives, heartburn, headache and urinary incontinence (particularly elderly women). Rare complications include soft-tissue (muscle, tendon, ligament, **fascia**) strain, chest discomfort, flushing, fall in blood pressure and delayed onset muscular soreness.

Recommendations

If possible, try to get an exercise program individually designed for you by a practitioner who has expertise in exercise therapy and who can take a full medical history and perform a physical examination including orthopaedic and functional testing. If you have any serious conditions, always seek approval from your therapist prior to starting any exercise program.

Proof of effectiveness

A systematic review found exercise therapy may be helpful for chronic low back pain in that it hastened return to normal daily activities and work. Exercise therapy that consists of individually designed programs, including stretching and strengthening, and is delivered with supervision can improve pain and function.

To stretch or not to stretch: that is the question

The practice of static stretching to prevent muscle soreness began in the 1960s when scientists thought that muscle soreness was due to muscles unaccustomed to exercise going into spasm, a theory that has since been disproven. There are several methods of stretching, and some are more effective than others. One method is dynamic stretching. Dynamic stretching uses momentum and active muscular effort to stretch a muscle into an extended range of motion; however, the end position is not held. Dynamic stretching has been shown to be an effective technique for enhancing muscular performance. Walking lunges is an example of a dynamic stretch.

Interferential current (IFC)

Interferential current is a medium-frequency alternating current, modulated to produce frequencies of between 1 Hz and 150Hz. It delivers current through the skin via strategic placement of superficial electrodes around a painful, target area or over a spinal nerve root, which is thought to penetrate the skin more deeply and cause less user discomfort than TENS (see below).

Research in the United Kingdom has consistently reported that IFC is the most commonly used electrotherapeutic treatment in Britain and Ireland for physiotherapy management of patients with low back pain.

Treatment normally begins by exposing the skin over the area of pain. Superficial skin electrodes are then placed over the areas of pain or the targeted area before attaching them to the device. The device is then programmed to deliver current at constant or varying intensities over a period of 15 to 30 minutes, during which the provider will periodically inquire about patient comfort and may increase current intensity to maintain a steady stimulus. The theory of action for IFC is to temporarily reduce pain in one location by stimulating pain in another location.

Reasons to have this treatment
This treatment is appropriate for acute and chronic non-specific back pain, muscle spasm and pain that covers a large area.

Reasons this treatment might not be suitable for you
Avoid use over the front neck region, heart, across the chest, areas of abnormal skin sensation, abdomen if you are pregnant, or if you have a cardiac pacemaker, implanted defibrillator or any other implanted electrical device. Patients with venous or arterial thrombosis or inflamed varicose veins also need to avoid this treatment.

Treatment effects
This increases local blood flow, reduces inflammation, reduces pain, relaxes muscle spasm and increases transmission across the cell membranes, which help movement in and out of the cells, and thus promotes healing.

Positive attributes
Small portable units can be purchased and used unsupervised outside a clinic setting. However, clear procedure instructions provided by a practitioner should always be sought prior to use. IFC decreases tissue resistance so stimulation is less painful. IFC is more comfortable than TENS and stimulates tissues deeper than a TENS unit. IFC does not usually produce visible muscle contractions unless applied on high settings.

Negative attributes
IFC doesn't treat the cause of the pain. It may mask more serious problems or conditions. Few portable units are available. It can sometimes become a panacea or crutch. Treatment focused on pain may psychologically reinforce an abnormal cycle of pain behaviour or indirectly entice patients to take a less active approach to pain management, which may hinder progress toward fuller functional recovery.

Side effects
These include minor skin irritations. Skin burns are a rare occurrence and are generally associated with the inappropriate use of the machine, such as prolonged or continuous use, or incorrect placement or settings.

Recommendations

The electrode size and positioning is important. Persevere with this therapy if pain relief is not immediately obtained. Caution should be taken if using IFC while driving or operating heavy machinery.

Proof of effectiveness

Interferential current therapy combined with other interventions was shown to be more effective than placebo application at the three-month follow-up in subjects with chronic low back pain. Interferential current therapy included in a multimodal treatment plan seems to produce a pain-relieving effect in acute and chronic musculoskeletal painful conditions compared with no treatment or placebo. When IFC is used as a stand-alone treatment, its effect does not differ from placebo or other interventions (such as manual therapy, traction or massage). It has been found that for patients with acute low back pain there is no difference in the effects of SMT or IFC, whether used in combination or in isolation.

Kinesiology taping

Kinesiology tape or kinesio tape (KT) is a relatively new form of elastic bandage–therapy used in the treatment of athletic and other injuries. It can be used for injury prevention or during rehabilitation after an injury. The tape is a thin and stretchy elastic-cotton strip with a heat-activated acrylic adhesive. Kinesiology tape is a form of dynamic taping due to its ability to stretch, in some cases stretching to over twice its original length. If the tape is applied with more stretch than its normal length, it produces a recoil effect, which then creates a tension force on the skin and muscles on which it has been applied. The elastic property of the tape allows for greater range of motion than traditional rigid tapes, which often restrict movement. KT can be left on for longer periods of time (up to a week or more). The tape has similar properties to human skin in both thickness and elasticity, which means the tape doesn't bind or restrict range of motion, but still provides support and body proprioceptive input to the nervous system. KT is often used as an adjunct to other therapy and is rarely used as a stand-alone treatment.

There are several different manufacturers of kinesiology tape throughout the world and availability is country dependent.

Reasons to have this treatment

KT is good for bruising, fluid accumulation, inflammation, muscle activation and inhibition, instability, hypermobility, hypomobility, acute and chronic pain, injury prevention, poor circulation or healing.

Reasons this treatment might not be suitable for you

KT should be avoided when there is an allergic reaction to the tape or if there are severe injuries requiring greater support than the tape can provide. Taping that excessively restricts a joint's range of motion can lead to further injury. Taping should not be applied to lacerations, abrasions or blisters.

Treatment effects

The tape is designed to lift the top layer of skin off its underlying layer, increasing the space below, creating a negative pressure gradient and providing greater lymphatic drainage, which decreases swelling. The lifting of the skin is also said to take pressure off underlying pain-sensitive fibres and to stimulate **mechanoreceptors** (movement receptors) to improve joint proprioception. Better muscle endurance and increased performance is claimed with this therapy, as well as faster recovery after intense exercise.

Positive attributes

KT can be used as both an injury prevention and rehabilitative measure. The tape is latex free, making it somewhat hypoallergenic, and those with a hypersensitivity to latex can wear it. The tape is water-resistant and breathable due to the cotton fibres, which allow for evaporation, quicker drying and longer wear time. Taping has been proven to have a positive placebo effect; patients often feel safer or protected regardless of the physiological effects of the tape.

Negative attributes

The effectiveness of the tape is often dependent on its application, with novice tapers tending to get less effective results due to inappropriate placement. Patients can develop a psychological dependence on the external support. Incorrect taping might predispose to injury or cause severe blisters.

Taping is comparatively more expensive for injury prevention than other techniques such as bracing due to the need for continual reapplication.

Side effects
Common adverse effects include chafing or rash due to allergic skin reaction. Rare adverse effects include severe skin lesions or wounds or both.

Recommendations
Special care should be taken when applying the tape if you have a neurological problem involving sensory loss. Skin preparation should be carried out before taping. This includes the removal of hair, cleaning of skin, addressing of any lesions with necessary consultation, using adherents and avoiding the application of oils or creams.

Proof of effectiveness
Studies have shown that, when applied to the lumbar muscles of chronic low back pain sufferers, kinesio taping leads to pain relief and improved lumbar muscle function. A small improvement in strength and range of motion has also been demonstrated.

Massage therapy

When something is sore it is our natural instinct to rub or massage the sore area in an attempt to reduce the painful sensation. Massage in its most basic form is a way of easing pain, while at the same time aiding relaxation, promoting a feeling of wellbeing and a sense of receiving good care. The English word massage is derived from the Arabic word *mass'h*, which means to 'press gently'. Eastern cultures believe that massage has powerful analgesic effects, particularly if applied to the many acupuncture points of the body.

Massage is a very popular form of alternative therapy—in fact, a study showed that of all the alternative therapies used by rehabilitation patients at a New York medical clinic, massage was the most commonly cited form of therapy. Massage is commonly used by massage therapists as a stand-alone treatment; however, it can be employed as an adjunct to prepare the patient for exercise or other interventions.

Massage is thought to be clinically effective at providing symptomatic relief of pain through physical and mental relaxation, and thereby increasing the pain threshold through the release of endorphins.

Despite all the evidence on massage there continues to be a lack of understanding of how manipulation of soft tissue causes relief from a broad range of symptoms. Researchers suggest that further studies are needed to figure out precisely how massage works.

Tight muscles do not always need to be stretched

A very common and misguided concept is that if something is tight, it needs to be stretched. In some cases stretching can actually exacerbate the condition or symptoms. Studies have shown that muscles don't actually elongate (stretch) during a stretch. What occurs is that your body gets used to the pain of stretching, thus your muscles' threshold for pain simply increases. Thereafter, your joint's range of motion can go further once your pain threshold increases. The odd thing about stretching is that it is so entrenched into conventional thinking that people will continue to stretch even though they are getting no results whatsoever.

The most commonly applied therapeutic massage is known as 'Swedish' massage. There are several components of massage including effleurage, pétrissage, tapotement, friction massage and acupressure:

- **Effleurage:** the therapists' hands glide over the patient's skin overlying the muscles being treated. Oil or powder is used to reduce friction and continual hand-to-skin contact is maintained throughout the session. Effleurage can be superficial or deep. The main mechanical effect of effleurage is to displace fluid in front of the hands.
- **Pétrissage:** this involves compression of underlying skin and muscle between the fingers and thumb of one or two hands. Tissue is gently squeezed as the hands move in circular patterns perpendicular to the direction of the compression. The manual compression and subsequent release causes the physiological effect of increased reactive circulation.
- **Tapotement:** this is a percussion form of massage that involves the use of both hands to repetitively strike soft tissues in a gentle, rapid and rhythmic fashion. There are many variations of this form of massage.

The physiological effect is believed to result from compression of trapped air that occurs on impact.

- **Deep friction:** pressure is applied with the ball of the therapist's thumb, fingers or the elbow to work a patient's skin and muscles. Deep pressure avoids over-stretching superficial tissues by bypassing them and attempting to direct the forces to the deeper tissues of the body. Deep friction massage is most commonly used to prevent or break down scar tissue and adhesions.

- **Acupressure:** this is a traditional Chinese medicine technique derived from acupuncture. It is a form of touch therapy whereby physical pressure is applied to the acupuncture points of the body using the hands, elbows or with various devices. Imbalances along the energy meridians are believed to cause disease and can be rectified using localised pressure.

Reasons to have this treatment
Massage is good for muscle soreness and stiffness, decreased range of motion, relaxation, pain management, poor circulation, non-inflammatory arthritis, lymphatic drainage and fluid retention.

Reasons this treatment might not be suitable for you
Avoid massage over tumours, open wounds, infected tissues, burns, nerve entrapments, deep vein thrombosis, severe varicose veins, non-consolidated fracture, severe clotting disorders or if on large doses of anticoagulant drugs or with inflammatory conditions (gout, rheumatoid arthritis and cellulitis).

Treatment effects
Massage has mechanical and psychological effects. Reflexive effects include dilating the blood vessels and so improving circulation, general relaxation, increased perspiration and a reduction in pain by way of releasing feel-good hormones and regulating neurotransmitters. Mechanical benefits include increasing lymph drainage, assisting blood flow, decreasing muscle tightness, preventing or breaking adhesions in soft tissues and softening scars. The psychological effect is 'the laying of hands' promotes a general sense of wellbeing and being personally cared for.

Positive attributes

Massage is widely available, inexpensive and effective for low back pain. Most people find massage to be relaxing and enjoyable. Massage can be used for relaxation on asymptomatic individuals without pain or problems.

Negative attributes

There are numerous massage techniques, which can be confusing for people, particularly if they cannot recall the massage technique they previously received. Practitioners often differ widely in the force and pressure being applied during treatment; some techniques require greater force while others require only minimal force. Although generally positive, the effects can be short-lived.

Side effects

Common adverse effects include soreness during or after treatment and allergic reaction (rash or pimples) to the massage oil. Rare adverse effects include worsening of presenting pain or minor soft-tissue damage. Rare complications include poisoning of the kidneys by the waste products of an injured muscle.

Recommendations

You should communicate with the practitioner during each session. At the start of the treatment session, you should advise the therapist of any areas you would like worked on as well as areas that should be avoided. How firmly the massage is to be applied needs to be discussed before commencement. If you feel the therapist is touching you inappropriately or is making you uncomfortable during treatment, ask them to stop immediately or ask them to work on another area. However, it should be recognised that massage treatment for low back pain often involves massage of the buttocks and sometimes the tailbone region.

Proof of effectiveness

A systematic review concluded that massage may be of benefit for patients with subacute (lasting four to 12 weeks) and chronic (lasting longer than 12 weeks) non-specific low back pain, especially when combined with exercises and education. The amount of benefit was more than that achieved by joint mobilisation, relaxation, physical therapy, self-care education or acupuncture. Acupressure or trigger point massage techniques seem to provide more relief than classic (Swedish) massage, although more research needs to happen to confirm this.

Scar tissue

This is a type of fibrous adhesion often referred to as 'fibrosis'. It develops due to a lack of oxygen at the cellular level (**hypoxia**); the body misinterprets this symptom as a signal to repair the oxygen-deprived tissues. A proliferation of repair cells, called fibroblasts, ensues, which try to repair the area by laying down new tissues; however, this only leads to the formation of scar tissue and adhesions within and in-between tissues. Scar-tissue formation can lead to reduced range of motion, muscle weakness, pain, compensatory movement patterns or neurological symptoms if a nerve becomes entrapped.

Interestingly, recurrent muscle tears tend to occur in the muscle tissue next to the old tear. Scar tissue is arguably the most common and most easily reversible condition of the musculoskeletal system.

Myofascial release

The word **myofascia** denotes the inseparable nature of muscle tissue (myo) and its accompanying connective tissue (fascia). As discussed in Chapter 1, unfortunately fascia was ignored in the past and was regarded as a useless packing tissue of the body. Fascia is now being vigorously studied. Despite previous neglect, myofascial therapies have existed for a few decades. Myofascial release is a hands-on or instrument-assisted soft-tissue therapy that can directly change and restore the health of myofascia within the body. Instrument-assisted soft-tissue mobilisation (IASTM) was formally introduced in 1994. Currently there are many myofascial techniques; below is a short list and description of some of the more popular techniques available.

Active release techniques (ART)

ART is a manual hands-on myofascial release technique that was developed by an American chiropractor, Michael Leahy, in the early '80s. It has now become one of the most popular forms of myofascial release techniques. The technique involves the practitioner taking the patient's tissue from a shortened position to a fully lengthened position while the contact hand holds tension longitudinally along the soft tissue fibres and the lesion, which effectively breaks down adhesions or scar tissue.

Fascial manipulation

This is a manual therapy for the treatment of musculoskeletal pain developed by Luigi Stecco, an Italian physiotherapist. The method has been developed and refined over the past 30 years through anatomical studies and clinical practice; it is based on a three-dimension biomechanical model for the human fascial system.

Guā Shā

Guā Shā is a traditional East Asian technique; it involves the use of a smooth-edged instrument to unidirectionally press-stroke the body's superficial tissues to create transitory therapeutic petechiae called 'sha'. Petechiae are small red spots of blood in the skin created by this therapeutic pressure. These represent extravasation of blood beneath the skin and fade in two to three days. Guā Shā has been used for centuries in Asia as a form of self or familial care in the home. Traditional tools include a soup spoon, coin, honed horn, bone, jade or stone. This treatment should not be attempted at home without expert guidance.

Graston technique

This incorporates the use of patented stainless steel tools with a unique curvilinear treatment edge, contoured to fit various shapes of the body and used to treat soft-tissue dysfunction. The technique is a comprehensive approach that, based on examination and findings, integrates IASTM with a rehabilitation program, including targeted stretching and strengthening exercises. Mechanical load-producing fibroblastic proliferation and the creation of new collagen is believed to be the reason for the effectiveness of friction massage and IASTM.

Reasons to have this treatment

Myofascial release decreases myofascial adhesions or scar-tissue formation, muscle soreness and stiffness, and helps with tendon disorders, distorted myofascia, decreased range of motion, pain management, poor circulation, non-inflammatory arthritis, lymphatic drainage and fluid retention. It also helps with acute and chronic non-specific mechanical low back pain and nerve entrapments.

Reasons this treatment might not be suitable for you
Treatment is to be avoided over tumours, open wounds, infected tissues, haematoma, burns, deep vein thrombosis, severe varicose veins, recent fractures, and on patients with severe clotting disorders, those experiencing fever or on large-dose anticoagulant drugs. This is not suitable for patients with inflammatory conditions (gout, rheumatoid arthritis and cellulitis).

Treatment effects
It is believed that these techniques repair degenerated tissue by introducing a controlled amount of microtrauma and re-initiating the inflammatory (healing) process.

Positive attributes
The use of soft-tissue instruments such as Graston technique or Guā Shā are especially effective in determining the direction of myofascial barriers. Most myofascial release therapies provide some instantaneous results; patients should be able to notice a measurable improvement in function or a decrease in symptoms at the end of each treatment session.

Negative attributes
Treatment is generally uncomfortable and can even be painful, particularly in those with long-term problems.

Side effects
Common adverse effects include soreness after treatment. Bruising sometimes occurs; it is not a desired effect but should not be a problem in healthy individuals. With traditional Guā Shā, red marks (petechia) are not an adverse effect; it is the intended effect.

Recommendations
If you do not notice some improvement within a few treatment sessions, try a different therapy. IASTM tends to be effective only for superficial

myofascia, while hands-on myofascial release techniques work better on deep fascial areas. Therapists should try to avoid using excessive force or over working one particular area in an effort to minimise adverse effects of treatment such as bruising.

Proof of effectiveness
Studies have found that patients treated with myofascial release showed a reduction of pain and improved function, less disability and increased mobility.

Spinal manipulative therapy (SMT)

SMT is a 'hands-on' therapy whereby a spinal joint is either mobilised or manipulated. Mobilisations use low-speed, passive movement techniques within the patient's range of motion and control. Manipulation is a high-speed, low amplitude, thrust at or beyond a spinal joint's physiological barrier, which often results in an audible 'crack' sound—otherwise known as a **cavitation**. Despite the fact that SMT has been used by osteopaths and chiropractors for over a hundred years, we still don't understand all the mechanisms and physiologic effects of this therapy.

Joint manipulation

Ever wonder what that crack sound is when a joint is manipulated? Most moving joints of the body are **synovial joints**. That is, they have two articulating bones separated by a cavity that is filled with synovial fluid and surrounded by a **joint capsule**. The synovial fluid contains dissolved gases such as oxygen, nitrogen and carbon dioxide. When a synovial joint is manipulated the sudden pressure drop within the joint causes a rapid release of these gases, which forms bubbles. The noise created by this gas release causes a 'cavitation', which is the term for that cracking sound. After a joint has been cavitated it cannot be cavitated again until the gases have seeped back into the joint fluid, which normally takes 20–30 minutes.

Many practitioners such as chiropractors, osteopaths, manipulative physiotherapists and orthomanual therapists (medical doctors trained in manipulative techniques) use SMT in day-to-day practice for the treatment of back pain. Most general practitioners have neither the time nor inclination to master the art of manipulation and may wish to refer back pain patients for this therapy.

SMT has been found to be at least as effective as other therapies such as physical therapy, analgesic use, exercises and back school, and significantly more effective than having no treatment.

Reasons to have this treatment

SMT is good for acute and chronic non-specific mechanical low back pain, and disc and nerve root problems such as sciatica.

Reasons this treatment might not be suitable for you

Absolute contraindications include active inflammatory arthritis, bone mineral deficiency, loose or dislocated ligaments, tumours or metastases, spinal infection, acute fracture or dislocation, acute spinal cord pressure and cauda equina syndrome. Relative contraindications include known malignancy history, benign bone tumour, spinal trauma, spinal hypermobility, history of spinal surgery, acute soft-tissue injury, blood and bleeding disorders. Disc herniation is sometimes listed as a contraindication to SMT; however, many manipulative therapists successfully treat disc herniation using SMT.

Treatment effects

SMT increases range of motion, increases pain tolerance or its threshold and improved nervous system coordination. Manipulation breaks up minor scar tissue formations and frees trapped joints. Several clinical trials indicate that spinal manipulation positively affects primary nerves from tissues surrounding the spine, the motor control system and pain processing.

Positive attributes

SMT is very safe, available and relatively inexpensive when compared to many invasive treatments. Good results are usually obtained in a short amount of time.

Negative attributes

There are some potential adverse effects after treatment. Some back conditions are not responsive to SMT. Certain patients may be fearful of SMT due to the physical nature of the treatment. Minor post-treatment soreness is a common but benign effect after a treatment. In rare instances, manipulation may make some patients worse.

Side effects
Common side effects include local discomfort, headache, tiredness and radiating discomfort. Complications of thoracic and lumbar spinal manipulation are rare. Exacerbation of the existing condition sometimes occurs. Cauda equina syndrome, lumbar pedicle fracture, lumbar/thoracic compression fracture, rib fracture, lumbar/thoracic disc herniation. The frequency of cauda equina syndrome has been estimated to be one in several million treatments.

Recommendations
You should always consider SMT before having low back surgery. It is relatively safe and serves as a good starting point in conservative care. SMT should at least be looked at before progressing to any of the more invasive therapies.

Proof of effectiveness
A recent high quality study found that when SMT was combined with exercise it is more effective than SMT alone, exercise alone, or physician consultation alone.

Is it OK to 'crack' myself?
Answer: no. The problem is that when patients 'crack' (cavitate) their neck or back by virtue of twisting, pushing or pulling their spine one way or another, they usually succeed in only manipulating joints that are already too loose. Generally this provides only temporary relief as the body will attempt to stabilise the now hypermobile vertebrae, which the patient interprets as a stiffening of the neck or back. Continual self-adjusting perpetuates the condition and can lead to excessive wear of the hypermobile joints. A better solution is to see a practitioner who is trained in a spinal manipulative technique, who will effectively identify the dysfunction and correct the appropriate

joints. This will result in better and longer lasting results. After treatment, patients often notice increased range of motion, reduced muscle tightness and a decreased desire to 'crack' themselves.

TENS

Transcutaneous electrical nerve stimulation (TENS) delivers an electrical current through superficial electrodes placed on the skin around the affected area, causing a tingling sensation and disrupting the pain signal in surrounding nerves. There are a few different electrode placement procedures based on the desired effect: around or near the lesion site, along the course of the peripheral nerve carrying the pain messages, on the back or at related acupuncture points.

Treatment normally begins by exposing the skin over the patient's area of pain or target area, which may be cleaned by the provider. The surface electrodes are then placed over areas of pain or the targeted area before attaching them to the device. Then current intensity is gradually increased until a tingling sensation is produced. The device is then programmed to deliver current at constant or varying intensities over a period of 15 to 30 minutes.

TENS is used by a wide variety of therapists. Patients can purchase their own personal portable TENS machine that they can use in a home setting.

Reasons to have this treatment
TENS is used for acute and chronic back pain, myofascial pain, arthritic pain, post-amputation phantom limb pain and pain due to peripheral neuropathy.

Reasons this treatment might not be suitable for you
Avoid treatment over the front neck region, heart, across the chest, areas of insensitive skin, abdomen of a pregnant woman, patients with a cardiac pacemaker, implanted defibrillator or any other implanted electrical device, and for patients with venous or arterial thrombosis or thrombophlebitis (inflammation of veins).

Treatment effects
TENS stimulates nerve fibres for the symptomatic relief of pain. Pain relief is based on jamming the incoming sensory pain signals.

Positive attributes

Small portable units can be purchased and used unsupervised outside a clinic setting. However, clear procedural instructions provided by a practitioner should always be sought prior to use.

Negative attributes

TENS reduces the perception of pain, but not the cause of pain. It may mask more serious problems. Patients can become too reliant on it. There is a lack of research on TENS, which means researchers do not fully understand it yet. Treatment focused on pain may psychologically reinforce an abnormal cycle of pain behaviour or predispose patients to take a less active approach to pain management, which may hinder recovery.

Side effects

TENS can cause minor skin irritations. Skin burns are a rare occurrence and are generally associated with the inappropriate use of these interventions, such as prolonged or continuous use, or incorrect placement or settings.

Recommendations

If you wish to try TENS, only do so as an adjunct for immediate to short-term pain relief. The outputs of electrostimulators must be calibrated and you must be adequately trained to use these devices safely.

Proof of effectiveness

Significant clinical effectiveness for TENS in the management of pain associated with osteoarthritis has been demonstrated. A number of studies show that TENS may be a useful adjunct to other treatments.

ENAR

A relatively new electrotherapy device in some ways similar to TENS is the electro neuro adaptive regulator (ENAR). Having wide applications, the ENAR appears to be especially useful in the treatment of pain syndromes. A randomised controlled trial on chronic neck pain sufferers found significant decreases in pain levels and improvement in function. Further research is required to better understand the scope and efficacy of this device.

PENS

Percutaneous electrical nerve stimulation (PENS) is a form of electro-analgesic therapy that provides non-drug analgesic therapy by combining the benefits of TENS and electroacupuncture (electrical stimulation at specific acupoints via needles placed in the skin).

PENS is comprised of a low-voltage pulse generator (TENS) device that is connected to two acupuncture needles through which a small electric current is passed. The therapy involves the placement of acupuncture needle probes in the soft tissues or muscles to stimulate peripheral sensory nerves at the sites corresponding to the local problem. This may generate a sensation of tingling and muscle contraction. The duration of treatment varies but each session typically lasts between 15 and 60 minutes.

PENS focuses on the treatment of pain, meaning needle electrodes are generally only placed at the site of local pain. It is believed that PENS can augment the effects of traditional acupuncture, can restore health and wellbeing, and is particularly good for treating pain.

Reasons to have this treatment
This helps with acute and chronic back pain, myofascial pain, arthritic pain, sympathetic nervous system–mediated pain, neurogenic pain, visceral pain, diabetic neuropathy and post-surgical pain.

Reasons this treatment might not be suitable for you
PENS should not be performed over the front neck region, carotid sinuses, heart, across the chest, areas of insensitive skin or the abdomen if a patient is pregnant. It should not be used on a person with a pacemaker, implanted defibrillator or any other implanted electrical device, and it is not suitable for patients with venous or arterial thrombosis or thrombophlebitis. Patients who fail to comprehend the therapist's instructions or who are unable to cooperate should not attempt this therapy. Skin areas affected by a dermatological condition such as eczema or dermatitis may not be suitable either.

Treatment effects
PENS causes the release of naturally occurring opioids such as ß-endorphin which generally produces pain relief for up to two hours.

Positive attributes

PENS can provide effective short-term pain relief. The PENS device is relatively inexpensive and widely available. It avoids the potential side effects related to the use of analgesic medications, and it can decrease the need for other more invasive procedures.

Negative attributes

Prolonged PENS appears to cultivate a tolerance to the pain-relief effect, making it less and less effective over time. The number of treatment sessions and the period of treatment required to sustain pain relief after therapy are unclear. Currently no studies have demonstrated PENS to be effective at producing any long-term pain-relief effects.

Side effects

Electrostimulator devices emit enough current to lead to tissue damage, electrolysis and electrolytic degradation of the acupuncture needle.

Recommendations

Ensure the outputs of electrostimulators are calibrated and that you are adequately trained to use these devices safely. Otherwise seek a referral for an experienced therapist to deliver this therapy.

Proof of effectiveness

Two randomised controlled trials of PENS therapy demonstrated short-term benefits in patients with chronic low back pain secondary to osteoarthritis and degenerative disc disease. Repeated PENS has been found to be more effective than TENS for chronic low back pain.

Therapeutic ultrasound

Therapeutic ultrasound (US) produces sound waves transmitted to the affected area through a handheld probe using conductive gel, thought to penetrate deep tissues and improve healing. Unlike US employed for imaging purposes, therapeutic ultrasound has a one-way energy delivery. Therapeutic ultrasound is medically categorised as a physical agent because it produces heat. Unlike most other heating agents (heatpack, whirlpool, heat lamp), which can only cause surface temperature changes, therapeutic ultrasound can be used as a deep-heating agent that has been shown to cause temperature changes in tissue 3 cm or deeper through the conversion of non-thermal energy source into heat within tissue.

Therapeutic ultrasound is commonly used in three forms: continuous, for raising deep tissue temperature; pulsed, for activating non-thermal physiologic effects; and phonophoresis, which is a method of using US to transmit topical medication through the skin. Ultrasonic energy causes soft-tissue molecules to vibrate from exposure to the compression and rarefaction caused by the acoustic wave. Increased molecular motion leads to microfriction between molecules and generation of frictional heat, thus increasing tissue temperature.

The intervention begins by exposing and cleaning the skin over the painful or target area. A conductive gel is then applied to the handheld US probe and spread over the treatment area. The provider then slowly moves the US probe in circular motions over the target area during a specific treatment time, usually 6 to 10 minutes. Unlike TENS, EMS and IFC, patients may not feel US while it is being applied.

Reason to have this treatment
Continuous ultrasound has shown positive effects in the treatment of acute and chronic pain, scar tissue, joint contractures, tissue adhesions and abnormal shortening of connective tissue. Pulsed ultrasound is mainly used for treating acute and chronic inflammation.

Reasons this treatment might not be suitable for you
These include directing acoustic energy over plastic implants, haemorrhagic regions, cemented areas of prosthetic joints, infected lesions, electronic implants (including neurostimulators), areas that have been exposed to radiotherapy within the past six months, fractures, bone growth plates in children and adolescents, thrombotic areas, orbits of the eyes, gonads and spinal cord after back surgery. Avoid treatment over circulation-impaired areas, carotid sinus or the heart, pregnant abdomens, acute bone fracture, active haemorrhage, tumours and areas of decreased sensitivity. Patients with seizure disorders, those unable to report stimulation-induced pain and those with known allergies to gel or pads may not be suited to this treatment.

Treatment effects

Ultrasound is believed to cause increased collagen extensibility, increased nerve signalling speed, altered local blood flow, increased enzyme activity, alterations in muscle contraction activity and increased pain threshold.

Positive attributes

Pulsed ultrasound can be used for treating pain and inflammation via phonophoresis. Ultrasound can provide an opportunity to mobilise tissue or treat movement impairments by heat-induced changes.

Negative attributes

In order to neurologically interrupt pain transmission and provide pain relief, US must be applied to the specific source of pain generation. The therapeutic actions of ultrasound are almost exclusively at the tissue level and, therefore, are ineffective for central pain or chronic pain.

Side effects

Bone pain can occur from continuous ultrasound. Inflammation can happen in the area being treated. Poor coupling can lead to overheating of the applicator, which could damage the device or burn the patient or both. If any pain or an uncomfortable 'prickly' sensation is felt by the patient, this could indicate that the bones or nerve endings in the target area are becoming, or are already, overheated.

Recommendations

Therapeutic ultrasound should be used as an adjunct therapy, not as a stand-alone treatment. The probe needs to be continuously moving during treatment in order to maximise effect and minimise the risk of burns. Circular- or stroking-probe movement techniques are commonly used and recommended. A practitioner should be present during the entire treatment session, so the intensity can be reduced or the treatment can be terminated if the patient shows any sign of distress.

Proof of effectiveness

Ultrasound for pain relief has been used for decades but its value as a standalone therapy has not been proven. The best available clinical evidence is that therapeutic US can be a useful adjunct when used with other therapies.

Traction therapy

The goal of this therapy is to separate vertebrae to create more space for nerves where they exit the spinal column, or to relieve pressure on the intervertebral discs or facet joints. History reveals various forms of traction have been used for pain relief since as early as the time of Hippocrates. Despite this long history of use, its effectiveness has yet to be proven. Traction is a commonly used method to treat low-back pain and sciatica in the United States. Up to 30 per cent of physiotherapists in Ontario, Canada, use spinal traction for sub-acute low back pain and acute low back pain with sciatica.

The rationale behind traction is that it causes spinal elongation through an increase of intervertebral space and relaxation of spinal muscles. However, spinal traction is unlikely to reduce or stabilise a prolapsed or herniated disc or make an annular tear disappear. To date there is little evidence of how traction truly works. Many causes of low back pain can be directly or indirectly attributed to the effect of compression on spinal structures. Various types of traction are used in the treatment of low back pain, usually in conjunction with other treatments. The most common forms of traction for the treatment of low back pain are mechanical or motorised traction (where the traction is exerted by a motorised pulley) and manual traction (in which the traction is exerted by the therapist, using his or her body weight to impart the force and direction of the pull). Some traction units require the patient to lie face down while treatment is given; other units place the patient on their backs.

Traction can be applied intermittently or continuously. Intermittent traction is where the force of pull is used on and off. Continuous traction is when the force of pull is held for an extended period of time, usually no more than 30 minutes. There is controversy over the magnitude of force required for intervertebral separation; however, there is evidence to suggest that even a small force of 9 kilograms provides a mechanical effect. For the lumbar spine the amount of traction needed to begin genuine separation of the vertebrae is half the patient's body weight. Inversion tables are a form of traction that uses a person's own body weight and gravity to stretch the spine. Inversion tables can be purchased by anyone and used at home; however, approval from a practitioner should be sought first. Some forms of spinal manipulation apply traction very specifically, but this would be recognised as manipulative therapy rather than traction.

Manual traction of the lumbar spine only increases the height of each disc by approximately 0.1 mm, but this net gain is lost as soon at the patient stands up and gravity loads the spine.

Reasons to have this treatment
Traction therapy can help acute and chronic non-specific mechanical low back pain, spinal nerve root impingement, herniated lumbar disc, ligament encroachment, narrowing of the intervertebral foramen, **osteophyte** encroachment, spinal nerve root swelling, joint hypomobility, degenerative joint disease, extrinsic muscle spasm and muscle guarding, discogenic pain, joint pain and compression fracture (sub-acute stage).

Reasons this treatment might not be suitable for you
Traction therapy should be avoided if there is acute inflammation, strains, sprains, joint hypermobility, pregnancy, cauda equina syndrome, aortic aneurysms, hiatal hernia, active peptic ulcer, osteoporosis, inflammatory arthritis and spondylolisthesis. Some patients with respiratory problems or those with claustrophobia may be unsuited to this treatment if a restrictive harness is used.

Treatment effects
Proposed physiological effects include distraction or separation of the vertebral bodies, a combination of distraction and gliding of the facet joints, tensing of the ligamentous structures of the spinal segment, widening of the intervertebral foramen, straightening of spinal curves and stretching of the spinal muscles. Patients will experience some form of pain relief by decreasing the compressive forces being placed on the spine.

Positive attributes
Many variations of traction exist and there are many different protocols. Traction is widely available and relatively inexpensive.

Negative attributes
It is difficult to identify patients who may benefit from traction. Continuous traction has proven to be relatively ineffective and to often aggravate

patients' symptoms. The patient must be relaxed during treatment for intervertebral separation to occur. To facilitate patient relaxation, the treatment must not aggravate the condition, and the patient must feel secure and well supported. Excessive force can increase pain or cause injury. Many traction protocols require multiple sessions over several weeks.

Side effects
Side effects include increased pain, respiratory constraints while wearing the traction harness or increased blood pressure during inverted positional traction. Anxiety is a common side effect with inversion traction. Rare complications include nerve impingement with heavy traction.

Recommendations
A trial of traction and compression tests should be used to determine if you are a suitable candidate for traction before undergoing treatment. If the manual tests cause no pain or provides relief, you are probably suitable for traction therapy. Large traction forces (more than half of your body weight) should be avoided.

Proof of effectiveness
Results of a systematic review found that traction as a single treatment for low back pain was more effective than placebo, sham or other treatment. For patients with sciatica there is moderate evidence that continuous or intermittent traction is no more effective than other treatments. Another review concluded that traction is most likely to benefit patients with acute nerve root pain with concomitant neurological deficit. Spinal traction is rarely given in isolation and is often provided in combination with other treatment modalities.

The main finding in the literature is that there is a lack of high-quality studies on spinal traction, which makes it difficult to form any concrete conclusions regarding effectiveness of traction.

Trigger point therapy

Trigger points are hyperirritable spots in skeletal muscle that are associated with very tender knots in the muscle. The spot is tender when pressed and can give rise to referred pain, motor dysfunction, and other reactions. Pain caused by trigger points is usually referred to as a myofascial pain syndrome. Risk factors for developing muscle trigger points include inactivity, stress, anxiety, muscle injury and older age.

The most common methods of trigger point therapy include ischemic compression, spray and stretch, myofascial release, trigger point injections and dry needling. Trigger point injections normally use a local anaesthetic such as Lidocaine or Procaine.

Ischemic pressure involves applying heavy digital (finger or thumb) pressure on trigger points, sufficient to produce skin blanching. Nimmo's explanations of the pathophysiology of trigger points are still regarded as accurate and highly sophisticated over sixty years later.

Unfortunately, the study of trigger points has not been incorporated into medical education. Some physicians believe that most common everyday pain is due by myofascial trigger points and that ignorance of that basic concept could inevitably lead to false diagnoses and the ultimate failure to deal effectively with pain. Trigger points have been implicated in the cause of headaches, neck and jaw pain, low back pain, the symptoms of RSI and many other forms of joint pain mistakenly ascribed to arthritis, tendinitis, bursitis or ligament injury. Referred pain from trigger points can mimic the symptoms of many other medical disorders; however, few doctors even entertain the idea of there being a myofascial source. Doctors at pain clinics believe that trigger points are the primary cause of pain in most cases and at least a part of virtually every pain presentation.

There still remains some controversy over the existence of trigger points despite over 60 years of information. Here are a few facts regarding trigger points. Trigger points can be manual palpated (felt with fingers). They emit a distinctive electrical signal that can be measured by sensitive electronic equipment. Finally, trigger points have been photographed in muscle tissue by using an electron microscope. Trigger point release (ischemic pressure) is the only form of trigger point therapy we are going to examine in this book. For more information on other forms of trigger point therapy consult volumes one and two of Travell and Simons's textbook on the subject: *Myofascial Pain and Dysfunction: The trigger point manual.*

Reasons to have this treatment
Soft-tissue trigger points, myofascial pain syndrome, acute and chronic muscle pain, myofascial hypertonicity, joint hypomobility and tension headaches can all benefit from this treatment.

Reasons this treatment might not be suitable for you
Ischemic pressure should not be applied to tumours, open wounds, infected tissues, burns, nerve entrapments, deep vein thrombosis, severe varicose veins, recent fracture, severe bleeding disorders or patients on large-dose anticoagulant drugs and inflammatory conditions (gout, rheumatoid arthritis and cellulitis).

Treatment effects
The applied pressure causes a temporary blood-flow restriction followed by a resurgence of local blood flow upon release. This eases the targeted trigger point, which in turn decreases pain and muscle tension while increasing joint range of motion and strength.

Positive attributes
Trigger point release is fast-acting, non-painful, effective, inexpensive, can give recurring benefits and is widely available.

Negative attributes
Untrained and inexperienced therapists rarely deliver the full benefits of treatment, which can cause patients to believe the treatment is ineffective.

Side effects
These include pain at the site of the actual trigger point or within the referral pain zone during or after treatment, and a worsening of pain after treatment.

Recommendations
Try to find a therapist who is very experienced in this technique. Ischemic pressure requires a specific amount of pressure to be effective; too much or too little pressure will render the treatment less effective.

Proof of effectiveness

The consensus following research is that manual therapies have acceptable support in the treatment of myofascial pain syndromes and trigger points. Trigger point therapy is now a widely available treatment approach.

Invasive therapies

Here is a list of the invasive back interventions examined in this book:
- Microdisectomy, laminectomy and foraminotomy
- Spinal fusion
- Intradiscal electrothermal therapy (IDET)
- Chemonucleolysis
- Percutaneous oxygen-ozone injection
- Prolotherapy
- Nerve block
- Radiofrequency denervation
- Epidural injection

Microdiscectomy, laminectomy and foraminotomy

These surgical procedures are used in cases of nerve root pain to enlarge the space around the nerve root. They are typically used to treat patients with a herniated disc that has failed to respond to conservative care. The procedures may be performed separately but are usually combined. Discectomy involves removal of disc material, laminectomy involves the removal of a small portion of bone (lamina) overlying the nerve root and foraminotomy entails expanding the channel through which the nerve root passes as it exits the spine. In each case the aim is to relieve neural impingement and provide more room for the nerve to move freely and heal. Previously, microdiscectomies were only done as open surgeries; however, with the recent advent of keyhole surgical methods, microdiscectomy procedures have been developed that are minimally invasive. This surgery involves cutting fewer back muscles when compared to open microdiscectomy. The belief is that the minimally invasive approach should allow patients to recover more quickly because of less tissue trauma.

While once popular, spinal keyhole procedures are increasingly being abandoned. Minimally invasive spine surgery was initially proposed as a means of minimising disruption to orthopaedic and neural structures. Unfortunately, as this keyhole approach is very limiting to the surgeon, he or she may need to use multiple entry points to achieve the desired surgical correction. In such cases more damage can be created than if a more conventional approach was adopted.

Both open and minimally invasive procedures require the administration of a general anaesthetic and a local anaesthetic, which is injected at the site of the incision. Open microdiscectomy strips some muscle material off the back part of the vertebrae, while the minimally invasive approach splits (goes inbetween) back muscles to access the intervertebral disc. Both procedures take approximately two hours to complete, and both generally require a hospital stay of one to three days (assuming no major complications arise). However, minimally invasive microdiscectomy patients can sometimes be sent home the same day as the procedure. Oral narcotics are given to patients post-operatively after both types of procedures to help with pain. Pain relief, particularly leg pain relief, is usually experienced immediately following the procedure. Neural symptoms such as numbness or paraesthesia may take weeks to months to recover.

Reasons to have this treatment
Spinal surgery is an option for an intervertebral disc herniation that has failed to respond to six to twelve weeks of conservative non-surgical care. Importantly, patients must have leg symptoms (pain, pins and needles, numbness or weakness) associated with their condition—not just back pain. Immediate spine surgery is generally only recommended in patients with a sudden onset of bowel/bladder incontinence (cauda equina syndrome) or for those who have progressive neurological deficit, such as a developing paralysis.

Reasons this treatment might not be suitable for you
Having back pain without leg symptoms is a contraindication to these procedures. Having back pain for less than three months is usually also regarded as a contraindication to surgery. Systemic infection, osteoporosis and the presence of other significant diseases can make this procedure unsuitable.

Positive attributes

Microdiscectomy, laminectomy and foraminotomy procedures can leave all the joints, ligaments and muscles intact, which allows the patient to maintain normal spinal movement. Microdiscectomy can now be performed as a minimally invasive surgical procedure and some patients can return to normal levels of activity relatively quickly.

Negative attributes

If delayed for too long, the results of spine surgery are not quite as favourable, so it is not generally advisable to postpone surgery for those with worsening nerve symptoms. Approximately 5 to 7 per cent of the disc space can be removed using a **posterior** microdiscectomy approach, and most of the disc space cannot be properly visualised. Repeat procedures, known as revision microdiscectomies (microdisectomy done on the same disc more than once) have decreased success rates compared to the first operation. After having a second surgery, the risk of requiring further surgeries increases.

Side effects

Aside from the known complications of surgery in general, postoperative complications include disc re-herniation, nerve root damage, bowel/bladder incontinence and infection. A rare complication is an accidental durotomy, (cutting the dural sac which can lead to cerebrospinal fluid leaking), which occurs in 1 to 2 per cent of surgeries.

Recommendations

Only opt for surgery if you have tried several conservative treatments and have failed to have any symptom improvements after six to twelve weeks. During this period of conservative care, try at least three approaches before considering surgery. Get a second opinion by consulting at least two different surgeons before proceeding with surgery.

Proof of effectiveness

It has been found that both microdiscectomy and conservative treatment patients have similar outcomes, although microdiscectomy patients have a more rapid initial alleviation of pain. A study comparing minimally invasive microdiscectomy to open microdiscectomy for lumbar disc herniations found no differences between the two groups in terms of operative time, length of stay, neurological outcome, complication rate or change in pain levels.

Spinal fusion

Spinal fusion is a surgical technique that permanently joins two or more vertebrae together. It is essentially a 'welding' process and is considered a major surgery. It is a treatment option for conditions such as spinal fractures, unstable spondylolisthes and degenerative disc disease (DDD) that fail to respond to a minimum of six months of conservative care. It is also used to correct abnormal spinal curvatures such as lateral curvature of the spine (**scoliosis**) or excessive forward curvature (**kyphosis**). As well as any condition that causes extensive damage to the spine and requires spinal fusion stabilisation. Of these conditions, discogenic pain is perhaps the most controversial indication for performing spinal fusion.

The rationale for spinal fusion is to create joint fixation (arthrodesis) to prevent movement at painful joints or to correct joint deformities. Spinal fusion is one of the oldest surgical interventions for the treatment of discogenic pain. A spinal fusion may be performed alone or in conjunction with discectomy or laminectomy.

There are various surgical approaches that surgeons use to perform this procedure. Under general anaesthetic a bone graft is performed in order to provoke bone growth between two vertebral segments and create a fusion, which effectively stops the motion at that joint. The bone graft consists of supplementary bone tissue taken from the patient (normally from the pelvis), called autograft bone, or harvested from cadaver bone (allograft bone), or consists of manufactured (synthetic graft) substitute. The vertebrae are also fixed together with metal hardware such as rods, screws, plates or cages. This fixation prevents vertebral movement while the bone graft fully heals. The bone graft healing process typically takes between three and six months but can take as long as 12 months in some cases. Surgery generally requires three to four hours to complete, and a hospital stay of three to four days afterward. Selection of the most appropriate procedure for each patient will depend on the nature and location of the condition being treated.

Several factors are pivotal in order to achieve a successful result from a spinal fusion such as an accurate pre-operative diagnosis, a technologically adept surgeon and a patient with a reasonably healthy lifestyle (non-smoker, non-obese, not of advanced age) who is motivated to pursue rehabilitation and restoration of his or her function. Spinal fusion for gross instability conditions (such as unstable isthmic spondylolisthesis) tend to be more successful than surgery done for back pain alone.

Post-operative care after spine fusion is very important and can lead to the ultimate success or failure of the procedure. During the first few months patients should avoid high-impact activities that may place the bone graft at risk. Permanent restrictions are only required in select cases. Since the bone graft is living tissue, after the fusion has established itself, the bone graft tends to get stronger in response to the level of strenuous activity.

It is important to remember that a spinal fusion requires the surgeon to cut through several layers of muscle and fascia to get to the spine. This permanently alters the function of these tissues by leaving scar tissue within and around these important soft tissues. Thus, it is imperative to restore the function of the tissues in order to avoid inhibited movement in the affected spine area. This can be achieved by having post-surgical soft-tissue work and exercise. A manual therapist can help to break down scar tissue and adhesions left over from the surgery.

Patients should always consult a practitioner who is knowledgeable about post-surgical rehabilitation prior to beginning any form of exercise. If your practitioner is not qualified or seems to be unsure of how to effectively provide a tailored, specific post-surgical rehabilitation program, ask if they can refer you to someone who is. It is generally recommended to begin rehabilitation exercises as soon as possible following back surgery in order to minimise physical deconditioning, joint contracture and further joint range of motion restrictions. It is advisable to work with a physical therapist for at least four to six weeks after surgery in order to ensure proper exercise technique and safety. Research has shown that in order to maximise recovery, education regarding posture, body mechanics and back protection is also critical. In most cases a post-surgical back brace does not need to be worn unless inadequate spinal fixation was achieved. If a patient had chronic low back pain prior to the procedure, the surgery is unlikely to completely resolve all the pain and symptoms; however, a moderate improvement in either pain or function is expected. Recurrence of spine problems may occur at any time following surgery.

Reasons to have this treatment

This surgery can work for degenerative disc disease that limits a patient's ability to function and has failed to respond to conservative care. Unstable spondylolisthesis, severe scolioses, spinal fractures and spinal deformities.

Reasons this treatment might not be suitable for you

Back pain of less than six months does not warrant spinal fusion. Patients with systemic infection, osteoporosis and significant health risks such as diabetes may also be unsuitable.

Positive attributes

Relatively high success rate (greater than 67 per cent) compared to other invasive procedures.

Negative attributes

The cost of the procedure is high compared to other invasive treatment therapies. Recovery and rehabilitation time is substantial compared to other forms of treatment. The full fusion process typically takes 6 to 12 months after surgery. There is a permanent loss of spinal flexibility following spinal fusion; the degree of loss is dependent, in part, on how many vertebrae are fused.

Side effects and complications

Side effects include clinical failure, which means the patient still has back pain despite a successful procedure. If solid fusion is not obtained (non-union), further surgery may be necessary to re-fuse the spine. Chronic pain may occur at the bone graft harvest site. Rare complications include nerve damage, infection or bleeding, anaesthetic complications, cerebrospinal fluid leak, and failure of the fixation hardware. The vertebrae above or below the level of the fusion usually degenerate faster due to greater stresses being placed on them.

Recommendations
Only in rare cases should a three-level (or more) fusion surgery for pain be considered. Spinal fusion of more than two levels is rarely successful in providing effective pain relief because it removes too much of the normal motion in the lower back and places too much stress across the remaining joints. Factors that can negatively affect the outcome of spinal fusion include smoking, obesity, malnutrition, osteoporosis, chronic steroid use, diabetes or other chronic illnesses.

Proof of effectiveness
Research shows that two-thirds of patients who have spinal fusion surgery for disc problems report good or excellent results.

Dynamic stabilisation

This is an option for those trying to avoid spine fusion, but require some stabilisation of the spine. Dynamic stabilisation uses screws and rods, similar to a fusion, but these rods are designed to allow for limited mobility between each segment and between adjacent vertebrae. In this procedure bone grafting is not necessary, eliminating the risk of unsuccessful bone grafting, one of the complications of spinal fusion. However, as with spinal fusion, spinal degeneration is progressive and leads to accelerated breakdown of adjacent vertebrae. In Australia this procedure is no longer regularly used.

Intradiscal electrothermal therapy (IDET)

IDET is a fairly recent and advanced procedure whereby an electrothermal catheter (heating wire) that allows for careful and accurate temperature control is inserted into the intervertebral disc and heats it up from within, cauterising the nerve endings within the disc wall to stop pain signals. It is a minimally invasive outpatient surgical procedure designed to help sufferers of low back pain caused by annular tears or small herniations of the lumbar discs. The procedure requires approximately one hour to complete and uses a local anaesthetic and mild intravenous sedation. A hollow introducer needle is inserted into the painful lumbar disc with the help of guided X-ray technology. Then an electrothermal catheter is passed through the needle and into the back of the disc. The catheter tip is slowly heated up to 90° celsius for 15 to 17 minutes. The heat contracts and thickens the collagen fibres within the disc, causing closure of the tears and cracks. Tiny nerve endings within the disc are cauterised, making them less sensitive. The catheter and needle are removed and, after a short period of observation, the patient goes home. A lumbar support is worn for six to eight weeks, followed by a course of rehabilitation. Improvements frequently occur within a few days of the procedure, but can take from six to eight weeks to become apparent. Spinal surgeons and anaesthesiologists with a strong background in pain management are best suited to perform the procedure. While initially popular, this therapy is falling out of favour.

Reasons to have this treatment
IDET can work for chronic lumbar disc pain sufferers demonstrated by MRI, CT scan or discography who fail to respond to at least six months of conservative (non-surgical) care.

Reasons this treatment might not be suitable for you
IDET is unsuitable for severe disc degeneration, spinal stenosis, neurological symptoms, large disc herniations.

Positive attributes
IDET improvements include increased physical activity, improved sitting tolerance and decreased use of pain medication. IDET is a relatively safe procedure, and the risks and complications including disc-space infection and nerve injury are negligible.

Negative attributes
IDET may not eliminate the need for surgery at a later time if severe symptoms persist.

Side effects
Allergic reaction to anaesthetic may occur. There have been isolated case reports of disc herniation, cauda equina syndrome and vertebral collapse being caused by IDET surgery. However, other studies have reported no adverse events.

Recommendations

Before considering this therapy, more conservative treatments should be tried. As per all spinal surgeries, careful choice of therapist and adherence to the post-operative rehabilitation schedule is essential. Ensure that the disc is not severely damaged. If so, microdiscectomy would be a better option.

Proof of effectiveness

Currently there are no long-term studies available on IDET; however, one small short-term study demonstrated that 60 to 74 per cent of patients who received IDET had significant pain relief that was sustained at 16 months. IDET procedure appears to offer sufficiently similar symptom improvement to spinal fusion, but with decreased risk of complications.

Chemonucleolysis

This is a minimally invasive technique that involves the injection of active enzymes into the nucleus (centre) of damaged intervertebral discs. The active enzyme speeds up the breakdown of the nuclear matrix, releasing water. As a result, the bulging disc is effectively shrunk, which in turn may decrease the pressure of compressed neurological structures. The belief is that a small change in disc volume produces a large change in pressure.

Minimally invasive treatments were developed to minimise risk and complications associated with more invasive procedures while still providing good clinical results combined with a well-tolerated, low-cost procedure. A major aim of chemonucleolysis is that, as a minimally invasive technique, it can help relieve back pain symptoms without the need for surgery. Depending on the health status of the patient, it may take weeks or months for the patient to return to normal activity levels.

Reasons to have this treatment

Chemonucleolysis is good for internal disc derangement and for patients with disc-related pain that is unresponsive to conservation care. Patients unwilling or unable to undergo surgical interventions have this option available.

Reasons this treatment might not be suitable for you

Patients who are allergic to the injected dye, enzyme or anaesthetic cannot partake in this treatment.

Positive attributes

Chemonucleolysis is an effective procedure that does not compromise future open surgery. Chymopapain has been shown to have fewer side effects such as allergic reactions than collagenase. Fewer hospital recovery days are usually required compared to traditional surgery. The complications following chemonucleolysis with chymopapain have been reported to be significantly lower than those that can occur after a disectomy has been performed.

Negative attributes

Normally after chemonucleolysis, patients may experience moderate to severe back pain and spasms that last two to three days, or longer, after the procedure. Often patients are given prescription medicines to control pain during this period. There are several possible complications.

Side effects

Allergic reaction to the enzyme, anaesthetic or the dye used during the procedure, which can range from a simple rash with itching and localised swelling to a life-threatening reaction that leads to difficulty breathing and shock (anaphylaxis). It should be noted that these reactions have been minimised with doctors testing patients for allergic reactions using skin tests prior to the procedure. The rate of anaphylaxis with use of chymopapain is remote (around 1 per cent). Increased back pain and muscle spasm after the injection. Intervertebral disc space narrowing may also occur after chemonucleolysis. Aseptic inflammatory complications or chemical inflammation (discitis) can result.

Recommendations

Minimally invasive treatments should be considered only after a trial of not less than four weeks of conservative treatment has failed. For at least six weeks following the procedure, it is recommended to avoid long periods of sitting and repetitive bending, stooping and lifting.

Proof of effectiveness

Research shows that chemonucleolysis can be an effective treatment for carefully selected patients. One study found that 83 per cent of patients had excellent or good results following the procedure.

Oxygen–ozone injection

Oxygen–ozone (O_2–O_3) injection is a form of chemonucleolysis, categorised as a minimally invasive treatment for disc herniations. Ozone is an unstable form of oxygen with the symbol O_3. O_2–O_3 is the gas mixture used in this procedure where 1 mL to 3 mL is injected under guidance of a CT scanner or discography into the disc and 7 mL to 9 mL is injected into the paravertebral muscle surrounding the disc. Ozone is a natural disinfectant, thus the ozone injected outside the disc serves to limit the risk of infection. Furthermore, ozone has been shown to have anti-inflammatory and pain-relieving effects. The procedure is usually performed in a surgical theatre and is normally completed in fewer than 30 minutes and only requires a short hospital stay. The success rate of the procedure has been reported to be approximately 75 to 80 per cent.

The procedure is believed to work by drying up part of the herniated disc. By decreasing the volume of the disc it may be possible to reduce nerve-root compression. Disc shrinkage may also help to reduce venous stasis caused by disc compression of vessels, thereby improving local microcirculation and increasing the supply of oxygen. This effect positively influences pain as the nerve roots are sensitive to hypoxia (lack of oxygen).

Oxygen–ozone injections have been found to help reduce the size of disc herniations. The ozone has a direct effect on the nucleus, which is replaced by fibrous tissues over a five-week period.

Reasons to have this treatment
This procedure is indicated for internal disc derangement. Patients with disc-related pain that is unresponsive to conservation care should consider this option. Patients unwilling or unable to undergo surgical interventions may be amenable to this treatment.

Reasons this treatment might not be suitable for you
Patients who are allergic to the injected ozone are unsuitable.

Positive attributes

O_2–O_3 injection can be safely repeated if it should fail to produce results the first time. O_2–O_3 treatment has the advantage of being applied to patients with nerve-root problems when other injection treatments are not appropriate. The low cost of O_2–O_3 therapy make this treatment very cost effective compared to other injection methods. It is safer than more invasive surgeries such as laminectomy; by avoiding the spinal canal, the O_2–O_3 injection eliminates the risks of post-operative scarring linked to surgery, which is often responsible for recurrence of pain. O_2–O_3 injection has been reported to have the best cost–benefit ratio and lowest complication rate (<0.1 per cent) of the current minimally invasive procedures. The procedure can normally be completed in less than 30 minutes.

Negative attributes

Several possible adverse effects or complications have been reported (see below).

Side effects

Allergy or a reaction to ozone can be an issue. Lumbar pain and distension, lower extremities and buttock pain, impaired sensitivity in the lower limb and aggravation of symptoms are also risks. All these symptoms are either intermittent or spontaneously resolved within 24 hours of the procedure. The Italian Oxygen–Ozone Therapy Federation (FIO) performed 15 000 O_2–O_3 injections and reported no procedure-related adverse events.

Recommendations

Minimally invasive treatments such as O_2–O_3 injection should be considered only after a trial of at least four weeks of conservative treatment has failed.

Proof of effectiveness

Research has calculated that the success rate for this therapy is around 75 per cent in terms of both pain relief and return to normal activity. This is on par with the success rate for microdiscectomy.

Prolotherapy

Otherwise known as sclerotherapy or regenerative injection therapy, this treatment involves injecting ligaments with compounds such as dextrose (sugar) and lidocaine (anaesthetic), which are believed to help restart the healing process by causing acute inflammation in the area of injection. Prolotherapy has been used for over 50 years, but has recently resurfaced as a popular musculoskeletal therapy. The theory is that by providing glucose (nutrients) to the site of injury, healing and repair of a stretched or torn ligament/tendon can be achieved. The injection essentially tricks the body into initiating a new healing cascade. This promotes tissue repair or growth. The injection can be comprised of different compounds at different concentrations and dosages, but a common recipe is a 20 per cent dextrose solution (concentrated sugar fluid) mixed with saline (salt water) and a local anaesthetic.

Reasons to have this treatment
Joint instability due to ligament or tendon damage can be benefitted from this treatment. Chronic pain due to sprain, strain, ligament injury and osteoarthritis.

Reasons this treatment might not be suitable for you
Relative contraindications include lumbar central canal stenosis, recent cortisone injection in the same area and use of medications that may interfere with healing. Absolute contraindications include neurological signs such as loss of bowel or bladder function, or loss of sensation or movement in the legs. Other absolute contraindications include active infections, abdominal aortic aneurism or any illness that can prevent normal healing.

Positive attributes
This is a minimally invasive procedure. Average number of treatments is relatively low (four to six usually required). The effects are permanent—once a ligament/tendon has been regenerated due to the treatment, it will remain that way unless it is reinjured. Prolotherapy can help soft-tissue regeneration in tissues that were damaged years or even decades earlier.

Negative attributes

The injection process is painful and pain in the area of injection may come back a few hours later and can last from one to ten days. Patients with needle-phobia may not be able to undergo the treatment.

Side effects

There is a small risk of infection during needle insertion. Needle insertion may produce some minor bruising, blood collection, local and general reactions.

Recommendations

Patients who are regularly using anti-inflammatory medications will have to stop taking them for several days after an injection.

Proof of effectiveness

A recent study concluded that for chronic non-specific low back pain sufferers, injections into ligaments, regardless of the injected solution, resulted in significant and sustained reductions in pain and disability. A 2010 systematic review found that in three studies, prolotherapy injections alone were not an effective treatment for chronic low back pain. They found that a combination of prolotherapy injections, spinal manipulation, exercises and other treatments can help chronic low-back pain and disability.

Another study found that prolotherapy was best used in conjunction with rehabilitative exercise.

Nerve block

A nerve block is a common injection procedure used for both diagnosing and treatment. Nerve blocks can be administered using various techniques, with the different methods of using nerve blocks depending on their location, the reason for the nerve block as well as the medical guidelines for their use. Examples of different locations include facet joint block, intradiscal nerve block, sympathetic nerve block, selective nerve-root block, and sacroiliac joint block. Research has repeatedly demonstrated that a diagnosis of the anatomical cause of back pain can only be reliably established if invasive tests such as nerve block are used.

Each procedure varies based on the involved anatomy; however, the basic approach remains quite similar. The procedure involves the injection of a steroid anti-inflammatory and a local anaesthetic (such as Lidnocaine) into or near the hypothesised pain generating tissue. Fluoroscopy (live X-ray) is used to guide the needle to the appropriate location. After the injection, the patient is monitored; if their pain is decreased by more than 50 per cent, it can be inferred that the pain-generating nerve has been identified. Following the injection, the steroid continues to have an effect by decreasing the inflammation around the injection site, which often aids in alleviating symptoms.

In cases of neural impingement it can occasionally be difficult to visualise which nerve is causing the patient's symptoms. In these instances a nerve block can be used as a diagnostic tool to figure out which nerve is being affected. In addition to its diagnostic function, this type of injection can also be used as a treatment for a far lateral disc herniation.

Reasons to have this treatment
Nerve blocks can be used diagnostically to determine the sources of pain as well as distinguish local from referred pain. Structures that can be diagnostically assessed using nerve blocks include facet joints, sacroiliac joints, intervertebral discs, nerve roots and sympathetic neural structures. Therapeutic nerve blocks are used to treat painful conditions such as nerve-root irritation, sympathetic nerve irritation, facet joint pain and sacroiliac joint pain.

Reasons this treatment might not be suitable for you
Nerve blocks may not be suitable for patients with drug allergies, blood clotting disorders or infection at the injection site.

Positive attributes
For selective nerve-root block, the injection is done outside the spinal canal, which eliminates the risk of cerebral spinal fluid leak due to a puncture of the dural sac (spinal cord sheath).

Negative attributes
Due to the use of fluoroscopy, patients are exposed to some ionising radiation.

Side effects

Occasionally the injection can temporarily exacerbate a patient's leg symptoms. Other possible complications include elevated blood sugars, rash, itching, weight gain, soreness at the site of injection and bleeding. Systemic toxicity of the local anaesthetic, nerve damage, damage to other structures around the injection site and local haematoma. Possible complications with facet nerve blocks include nerve damage, infection, blood-vessel injury, meningitis, punctured lungs, radiation exposure, facet joint injury and muscle bruising.

Recommendations

This procedure may be an option in cases where conservative therapy has not produced good results, yet the patient is unwilling to have surgery. Although there are currently no specific guidelines, it is recommended that patients receive no more than three injections per year.

Proof of effectiveness

While several papers report benefit, there are also reports that therapeutic nerve blocks for facet joints using intra-articular injection of steroids offer no greater benefit than injections of normal saline. Evidence of long-lasting success is lacking.

Radiofrequency denervation

This is a minimally invasive procedure and is also known as radiofrequency ablation, neurotomy, lesioning or rhizolysis. The procedure involves inserting a needle-sized probe into a patient who is lying down. The insertion goes through the back, which is positioned under fluoroscopic guidance onto the nerve supply to a facet joint. A local anaesthetic is injected into the region prior to the procedure and light sedation may be used. The probe has an electrode on its tip that is connected to a radiofrequency generator. This produces high-frequency alternating current that heats up the target tissue near the electrode. The current cauterises (burns) the selected nerves, which deactivates the pain-producing pathways. After the electrode is withdrawn, a small sterile dressing is applied to the injection site.

The procedure is commonly done on the **medial** branch nerves of the dorsal primary ramii, which supply the facet joints of the spine.

A local anaesthetic or steroid or both are injected after the probe has been removed to relieve discomfort following the procedure. The entire procedure takes approximately 60 minutes to complete. Patients are monitored for a few hours following the procedure before they are allowed to return home the same day.

The full benefits from the procedure may not appear until two to three weeks after the procedure. The nerves will eventually regenerate after the procedure, which usually takes between six months and two years, at which time back pain may or may not return. If it does, the procedure can be repeated.

Reasons to have this treatment
Thoracic and lumbar facet joint pain, sacroiliac joint pain and sympathetic system maintained pain are conditions suited to this treatment.

Reasons this treatment might not be suitable for you
Neurologic abnormalities, definitive clinical or imaging findings or both, proven specific causes of low back pain, including herniation, Grade 3 or Grade 4 spondylolisthesis, spondylosis, spinal stenosis, clinical **radiculopathy**, multiple sclerosis, coagulation disorders, pregnancy, metastatic cancer, infection and trauma contraindicate this procedure. Allergy to radiopaque dye or local anaesthetic, having more than one pain syndrome, lack of response to diagnostic nerve blocks and psychiatric disorders are also contraindications.

Positive attributes
Matching the right patient to this treatment is important for a good clinical outcome. It is a minimally invasive procedure and patients can go home the same day as the procedure—barring any complications.

Negative attributes
There is a lack of evidence to support the short-term effects of radiofrequency denervation for chronic low back pain.

Side effects
Common side effects include discomfort at the insertion site, transient burning pain, slight sensory loss, numbness, uncoordination and local

hypersensitivity. Rare complications include headache, blood tumour, infection at the injection site, allergic reaction to injected medication, new pain or worsening pain. Very rare complications include convulsions, temporary or permanent disabling nerve damage and cardiac arrest.

Recommendations

Diagnostic nerve blocks should always be performed before proceeding with radiofrequency denervation to ensure the suspected pain-generating tissue is indeed the source of the patient's back pain and to make sure the appropriate spinal level is treated. Be sure to tell your doctor about any medications you are currently taking, as well as any herbs, supplements and other non-prescription drugs, as these may exclude you from having radiofrequency denervation.

Proof of effectiveness

A study with a double-blind controlled design showed some effects in a small selected group of patients at three, six and 12 months after treatment, concerning not only reduction of pain but also alleviation of functional disability. There is conflicting evidence regarding the short-term effect of radiofrequency denervation on pain and disability in chronic low back pain of facet joint origin.

Epidural injection

The epidural space is within the spinal canal outside the dural sac, which contains the arachnoid mater, subarachnoid space, cerebrospinal fluid, the spinal cord and cauda equina (below the L1 vertebra). In humans the epidural space contains lymphatics, spinal nerve roots, loose fatty tissue and small blood vessels. The dural sac or dura mater is a covering that protects and insulates the delicate spinal cord and cauda equina within the spinal canal. The dural sac is very sensitive to compression or chemical irritation, both of that cause referral pain into specific areas of the back that correlate with the level of the compression/irritation.

Epidural injections are an invasive procedure and should be reserved for patients in whom conservative treatment has failed to provide adequate relief. Various drugs can be administered via epidural injection in an attempt to relieve back pain; these include morphine, steroids, saline and local anaesthetics or any combination of these drugs. The most commonly administered drug for the treatment of low back pain are corticosteroids. The rational for administering an epidural steroid for the treatment of low back pain is predominantly for the anti-inflammatory effect of the drug. Steroids inhibit the inflammatory response caused by chemical and mechanical sources of pain. Injections are usually performed in a surgery centre, hospital or a physician's clinic. Many types of doctors can be qualified to perform epidural injections including anaesthesiologists, radiologists, neurologists and surgeons.

The procedure begins with the patient lying face down on an X-ray table and a small cushion is placed underneath the abdomen to slightly curve the back. If the patient is uncomfortable in the prone position, the patient can lie on their side in a slightly curled position. Sedation is available if needed but is generally unnecessary. The skin in the low back area is cleaned and then numbed with a local anaesthetic. Using the fluoroscope for guidance the needle is inserted through the skin and directed toward the epidural space of the target level. Once the needle is in the proper position, the medication is slowly injected. Patients can feel a pressure increase in the area due to the volume of solution being injected, but it should not be painful. The procedure generally takes 15 to 30 minutes to complete. After the injection, the patient is monitored for 15 to 20 minutes before being discharged. Patients' back/leg pain may become worse for two to three days after the injection before it begins to improve. The steroids often take two to three days before patients begin to feel the beneficial effects.

Reasons to have this treatment
Epidural injections can be used in cases of lumbar disc herniation, spinal stenosis, vertebral compression fracture, annular tears and cysts that form in the facet joint or within the nerve root. Patients whose pain is not adequately controlled by less invasive treatments may also do well with this treatment.

Reasons this treatment might not be suitable for you
Epidural injections should be avoided when there is local or systemic infection as well as pregnancy (if fluoroscopy, a type of X-ray, is used). Patients

with bleeding problems—patients taking blood thinners (anticoagulants), patients with clotting problems (haemophilia)—and patients whose pain is due to a spinal tumour (if suspected an MRI scan should be done prior to the injection to rule it out) should not pursue this treatment.

Positive attributes

Presently most epidural injections are done under fluoroscopic guidance, which has been shown to improve the placement of the injection and reduce the risk of complications. Epidural injections deliver medication near or directly to the source of pain, providing fast relief. Normal activities can often be resumed the day after the procedure.

Negative attributes

Benefits seem to be of short duration only. Currently it is unclear which patients benefit from these injections. Controlled studies have found that medication is delivered to the wrong site in more than one third of epidural steroid injections performed without fluoroscopy. Currently there is no definitive research to provide guidelines on how many epidural steroid injections should be administered or how frequently they should be given.

Side effects

Common side effects include headache, dizziness, tenderness at the site of injection, tingling, numbness and nausea. Complications include nerve-root damage, infection in or around the spine (meningitis), bleeding around the spinal column (hematoma) and allergic reaction to the injected medication. Rare complications include cauda equina syndrome, paraplegia and paraspinal abscesses. Complications can vary depending on the approach of the procedure (lumbar versus caudal). An increased risk of infection exists with the caudal route, because of proximity of potential sources of infection.

Recommendations

Certain procedural guidelines can reduce the risk of complications and improve efficacy of the procedure. These include fluoroscopic guidance, prone positioning of the patient, and **lateral** injection at the relevant level and with a small volume of injectate as well as low-dose corticosteroid.

Seek out a doctor who is reputable and has extensive experience with epidural injections. Be sure to tell the doctor about any medications you are currently taking, as well as any herbs, supplements and other non-prescription drugs, as these may exclude you from having an epidural injections.

Proof of effectiveness
Many clinical trials have examined steroid injection therapy. Although there have been some encouraging findings, the research shows conflicting results. Therefore the value of epidural steroid injections has yet to be established.

Conclusion

It is important to point out that both invasive and non-invasive back therapies are constantly evolving and new ones are being developed every day. Procedures that are presently viewed as gold standards of treatment for specific back conditions may fall out of favour with doctors and be quickly replaced by refined procedures or new ones. We have deliberately avoided ranking the various therapies for this reason. Our goal is simply to explain the various options available when selecting treatment. Each patient is unique and, despite having the same diagnosis or clinical findings as others, each case of back pain is as unique as the individual.

Decisions regarding the optimal management of back pain are not easy to make. When confronted with the dilemma of choosing an appropriate treatment, you need to critically evaluate all the treatment options, consult with doctors, practitioners and specialists for their opinions, and come to a conclusion that best suits your needs.

There are many different options to treating back pain and it will be a process of finding the most effective therapy for your condition. Remember to always get a second opinion on any suggested invasive procedure, as a fresh pair of eyes can bring a new perspective.

My back pain story
Dan O'Brien

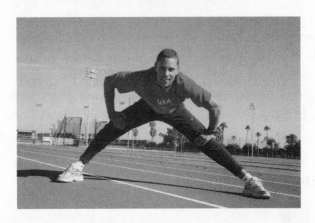

Despite being an Olympic champion and former world record holder in the decathlon, Dan achieved both of these goals with a broken back. Dan has had a break in his L4 vertebra his whole career.

In 1990 Dan was a track and field athlete in the decathlon when he began to experience frequent severe low back spasms. Dan went to his GP for help and was referred to a sports physician who promptly referred Dan for some spinal X-rays. The X-rays revealed that Dan had a spondylolisthesis of the L4 vertebra, which is a stress fracture (break) of the back part of the vertebra.

The specialist told Dan he had two choices: 1) stop doing athletics or 2) learn to deal with the debilitating back pain. Dan did not like those options, so he chose a third option—seeking out alternative methods for treating his low back, so he could continue to compete. A year into his search for an answer to his back pain, Dan met a chiropractor who manipulated his spine and managed to restore function and significantly reduce his back pain. Dan became much more aware of his body and he found that with regular chiropractic adjustments and massage, he was able to keep his back healthy and continue to train and compete in one of the most gruelling sports—the decathlon.

In his own words, Dan recounts an international decathlon competition in 1994:

'Sometime during the long jump (the second event of the decathlon) I felt my back go out and I could barely walk, let alone compete in eight more events. Luckily I had my chiropractor with me, and he adjusted my low back. Once I was adjusted, my back settled down and I regained full function, and went on to win the competition. My advice is find what works for you. Try different treatments or even different practitioners of the same method until you find the one that gives you the best results, and stick with them.'

Dan still gets some low back problems, but is able to keep his low back in working order by keeping up with regular core-stability exercises, stretching and functional exercises, as well as getting regular chiropractic treatments and massage.

5 How to choose a good therapist for your back pain

Why is having back pain so complicated? There's just too much going on. There are so many complex tissue types making up the spinal regions. Many things can go wrong. There are widely differing opinions on the true diagnosis in many cases. Once diagnosed, there is a huge variety of available treatment options. And, importantly, there are many different types of diagnosticians and therapists to choose from. In your case, more than one type of therapy or therapist may be necessary to adequately manage your back pain. Unlike most other diseases or disorders, back pain presents a real problem of choice.

Alternately, if you have a lung infection, high blood pressure or a broken arm, there are few choices about what needs to be done. Diagnosis wouldn't be difficult; the best person to manage your case and the appropriate treatment decisions would be relatively straightforward.

Let's have a look at the options you have in terms of finding the right type of practitioner for your particular problem—and how to find a good one.

The types of practitioners

The main groups of therapists are listed below. While many of them offer services other than just back care, we will only be discussing this aspect of their services.

Alternative medicine

This is an increasingly popular branch of health care that includes a variety of practitioners who focus on a range of approaches such as natural medicines, nutrition, exercise and eastern medicines. The quality of training of alternative medicine practitioners ranges from excellent to dubious and, apart from Traditional Chinese Medicine and acupuncture, in most jurisdictions in Australia these professions are not government-regulated. Therefore, greater care needs to be exercised in seeking out a good alternative-medicine therapist. Of all the alternative-medicine professions, to date only acupuncture therapy is well evidenced in terms of having proven effectiveness supported by research. Massage is also a well-researched therapy and has been found to have positive but usually only short-term effects. While therapeutic massage is popular with back pain sufferers, it is inadequate as a stand-alone therapy. For this reason we only recommend massage as an adjunct to other therapies. We believe that the other alternative-medicine approaches, such as massage or naturopathy, may be worth a try after you have exhausted other medical and complementary medicine options (see below). Other than acupuncture and massage, we can't recommend any other alternative-medicine approaches at this stage due to the lack of researched evidence to support their use in back pain care.

Complementary medicine and allied health professions

Approaches in complementary medicine and allied health are government-controlled by legislation and are taught in universities in Australia. Generally these therapies are widely accepted in our society. They tend to be well researched and there is fair to strong evidence of their value in the diagnosis and management of back pain. The main professional groups in this area are chiropractors, clinical psychologists, occupational therapists, osteopaths and physiotherapists. In this book we are differentiating treatment providers into three main categories: alternative, complementary (or 'allied') and medical. In the past, complementary and alternative medicine (CAM) therapists have been lumped together, but this is no longer appropriate as some of these therapies are government-recognised, publicly funded, and have some research evidence behind them. Others clearly do not have any of these features.

Chiropractors

These practitioners are well known for their management of back pain. Substantial research supports the effectiveness of chiropractic therapy for the management of mechanical back pain and some forms of nerve-root or disc-related back pain. Like the other professions listed below, chiropractic is a government-approved profession and all chiropractors are registered with the federal Department of Health. They are required to complete continuing education each year and comply with a code of conduct. Although they specialise in the use of spinal manipulation, chiropractors also employ many adjunctive treatments such as joint mobilisation, muscle and balance retraining, soft-tissue therapy and exercise rehabilitation.

Clinical psychologists

It is now widely accepted that people with chronic pain have significant psychological and social pressure placed on them. If these dimensions of their condition are not addressed, they will take longer to get better and have a more difficult return to normal function and employment. For this reason, most clinicians appreciate and adopt a 'biopsychosocial' approach in the care of their patients. Such an approach blends the anatomical, psychological and environmental components of back pain in coming up with effective management strategies. In this way, clinical psychologists have become a vital part of managing back pain cases, especially the more difficult and long-standing cases. They perform psychological assessments and deliver therapies including counselling, and cognitive and behavioural therapies.

Occupational therapists

These therapists aim to maintain the daily living and work skills of injured people. Treatment focuses on adapting the environment to the injured person's abilities, adapting the work tasks and educating patients. The primary goal is rehabilitation to enable people to participate in the activities of everyday life. Specifically, they may do the following:
- design and manage gradual return to work strategies
- educate people in safe work behaviours
- help change the work situation for individuals with special needs
- help prevent or minimise injuries.

They work in several settings, including hospitals, rehabilitation units, community health centres, psychiatric clinics, hostels, hospitals and private practice.

Osteopaths

In Australia osteopathy has developed along parallel lines to the chiropractic profession, making it difficult to find strong differences between these two types of therapists. Osteopaths also use spinal manipulation and mobilisation but tend to incorporate more soft-tissue therapies in their approach. They also commonly use muscle and balance retraining, and exercise therapy.

Physiotherapists

These practitioners diagnose and treat back pain and disability through physical means. Physiotherapists focus on movement and function to assist patients to overcome their back problems. They recommend exercise programs, sometimes use joint manipulation and mobilisation, re-educate muscles to improve control, and may employ massage, acupuncture and hydrotherapy as adjuncts. Electrotherapy (such as ultrasound) may be employed, but far less than it was used previously due to a lack of proven results. Like occupational therapists they can provide assistance with the use of splints, crutches, walking sticks and wheelchairs.

Medicine

In the medical profession there are three levels of practitioner who have an interest in back pain. They are general practitioners (GPs), musculoskeletal medicine practitioners and specialists.

General practitioners (GPs)

The first port of call for many back pain sufferers is usually their family doctor. Although it's natural to think of your doctor when you are sick, if you have a serious back complaint it shouldn't be managed by a GP alone unless he or she has a special interest in musculoskeletal medicine—such as a musculoskeletal medicine practitioner (see below). However, we recommend that you consult your GP to keep him or her in the loop and so that your medical history is up to date. Getting a recommendation from your GP on who to follow up with is also a good idea. But do it as soon as possible; if you have a back problem that is not trivial you need more focused care. Your GP can provide pain killers and anti-inflammatory medications, which can be a very important part of your care, but, when used alone, medications are very limited. Although they can provide symptomatic relief, they do little in terms of functional restoration or rehabilitation. These days, the level of diagnostic competence with a complex back diagnosis is high among the complementary and allied therapists so that the ongoing role of a GP in back pain care is limited.

Musculoskeletal medicine doctors

These are medical practitioners who specialise in physical medicine and rehabilitation. They combine physical therapies such as manipulation and exercise with the use of drugs, most commonly as injectables. If you wish to stick with a purely medical approach, this may be your best option. We suggest that you make sure that the practitioner is a member of a musculoskeletal medicine association and not just a GP with an interest in backs. We believe that when you have a back problem, you are best served by practitioners who make a genuine commitment to physical approaches, rather than jacks of all trades.

Medical specialists

Four types of medical specialist are important in the diagnosis and treatment of most spinal problems—neurologists, orthopaedic specialists, neurosurgeons and rheumatologists. While pathologists and radiologists are also consulted for diagnosis they do not provide therapy. Neurologists concentrate on the impact that the back problem has on the nervous system and use surgery and medications, and provide advice in their treatments. Orthopaedic surgeons are concerned with the mechanical aspects of the condition, and use surgery and drugs in treatment. Neurosurgeons specialise in surgical cases that involve the nervous system; they are often the specialists who perform back surgery in and around the spinal cord and nerve roots. Rheumatologists are most useful in the management of inflammatory conditions such as some forms of arthritis that can affect the back. They are diagnosticians, and use medications and provide medical advice.

As surgery is highly invasive and usually permanent, this strategy should be reserved as a last resort in your decision-making. Typically, surgery for back pain should not be contemplated within the first three months of experiencing a back problem. There are, however, some clear exceptions. If your back problem involves steady and progressive deterioration of function, or constant worsening of symptoms, then early surgery may be needed. The onset of loss of bowel or bladder function associated with a back problem may flag an emergency situation requiring immediate surgery.

Evidence-based medicine

The concept of evidence-based medicine (EBM) is now widely accepted as the best method of practice. The premise of EBM is that treatment decisions are based on a combination of three factors—the best current evidence, the practitioner's experience and the patient's preference. A practitioner who uses this philosophy diligently balances these three factors to tailor the best approach for each patient. This requires practitioners to constantly update their knowledge and skills in order to keep up with an ever-changing progressive process. This approach maximises your chance of receiving the safest and most effective care for your problem. It's in your best interests to consult practitioners who practice EBM.

Multimodal versus monotherapy

There is substantial evidence that back pain should be managed with more than one treatment approach (multimodal). This is best employed in a coordinated fashion, either by one therapist applying different types of treatment, or two or more therapists working together. Research on patients with back pain during pregnancy has shown that the combination of manual therapy (chiropractic) with standard obstetric care was superior to standard care alone in terms of pain relief and reducing disability. Another study conducted on patients suffering sciatic pain due to nerve-root compression found that they substantially improved after they were placed on a multimodal treatment plan. Adding the services of a clinical psychologist is valuable in multimodal treatment plans and, although known to contribute to better outcomes, it is not fully understood which components of the therapy have made a real contribution. However, not all studies have come to the same conclusion on the advantages of multimodal therapy. A further study found no advantage in a multimodal program over the use of exercise therapy alone.

Our advice is that if you don't obtain good results early on in your treatment, say within two weeks, you should ask your therapist to work out a multimodal program of care. Once started, you may be able to work out which components of the program appear to be most helpful and which may be dropped. As usual, make these decisions in conjunction with your therapist. If unsure, get a second or third opinion. Don't blindly follow advice no matter how confidently it has been given to you. Remember, it's your back and you are in the driver's seat, so don't be afraid to demand the care that you deserve.

Pills, needles and scalpels

These are the three most common methods of treatment in western medicine: oral tablets, needle injections and surgery. Notice that all of these options have been based around decreasing or eliminating the patient's pain. None of them addresses or is concerned with the cause of the pain; they only treat the symptom. It has been revealed that general practitioners prescribed analgesics (pain killers) to 80 per cent of patients presenting with back pain on their initial visit. Other options are available and if you haven't been advised about these options, you haven't been shown the whole picture. Don't be bullied into making a decision you are not sure about. Take your time and get informed—there may be a better option available that you don't know about. Be prepared to ask questions, especially if your expectations are not being met. You may need to either lower your expectations or ask about a different treatment approach.

Characteristics of an excellent therapist

Your first visit with any therapist should involve your evaluation of the therapist and a determination as to whether that person is right for you. We advise that you do your homework first. Read up on your symptoms and talk with your family doctor. The more you know about your situation, the better placed you will be to work out if a therapist seems to 'get you' or understands your case. Every patient is different and every therapist is different. You will get the best results from a therapist whom you appreciate and respect, and then you will be more likely to closely follow the advice that therapist gives.

There are four points you should consider when selecting a practitioner: knowledge, skills, attitudes and informed consent. Let's look at these factors and some pointers which can help you find the best therapists for you.

Therapist knowledge

While all therapists will have completed the required high levels of study and be suitably qualified and licensed to practise, obviously some will know a lot more than others about particular problems. In part, this is because therapists have differing areas of special interest—some may be more neurologically oriented or more capable with sports injuries or more focused on children's cases. On your first visit with a therapist, ask how often they treat your kind of problem, what they typically do and recommend for it. Please note that your practitioner may not be able to provide you with a diagnosis on your first visit. However, you should be wary if your practitioner fails to give you a diagnosis after several visits. Ask how long you'll be under their care and the factors that they believe will make your case an easy or difficult one to manage. If you've done your homework, you will be in a good position to judge how credible the therapist's responses sound to you.

Therapist skills

While it's impossible for you to fully judge the technical competency of a therapist, you can tell a lot by seeing how smoothly and competently your therapist physically handles you. You should look for a firm but gentle and confident touch. At all times your therapist should appear to know what he or she is doing and exude an air of being completely in control and well-coordinated as the situation progresses from history-taking to physical examination, to discussing your diagnosis and proposed therapy, and finally through to the delivery of the treatment. Any hesitancy, 'hmming and arring', and signs of not knowing what to do next should be obvious to you. They are an indicator that the therapist may not be the best for you or the management of your case. This may become especially clear when you are being physically handled. Some diagnostic tests and some treatments may be painful but, when performed by an expert, they are never unexpected, never uncontrolled, and should never leave you feeling apprehensive about your security.

Therapist attitudes

Finally, be perceptive of how your therapist greets you, communicates with you, and especially how well the therapist listens to you. The best therapists show genuine concern and a high level of interest in their patients. Even though they may have seen a particular kind of case hundreds of times, the best therapists approach each new patient with real interest and attention. Once again, this is because you are unique, and the individual characteristics of you and your condition deserve special attention. Be cautious of clinicians who seem not to be listening to you or who appear to be making their mind up before hearing your full story. There may be some clinicians who are easily distracted or allow interruptions that disrupt your consultation. Also, those who appear to be in too great a hurry should ring alarm bells— although you shouldn't confuse efficient, skilful, no-nonsense progress with someone who's just cutting corners. At the end of your session your therapist should explain their impression of your case to you. This should be clear and concise and should leave you feeling confident that they are on the right track. If your diagnosis is unknown, conservative and safe treatments should be followed until a clear diagnosis can be made. The therapist should also have a plan B in place in case your condition fails to respond to treatment.

Informed consent

Another good indicator of a professional attitude can be examined when your therapist informs you of their professional opinion and seeks your consent to proceed. We call this part of the consultation the 'gaining of informed consent'. This is a vital component of the doctor–patient interaction. This occurs when the clinician lays down the following information:

- the proposed tests
- the proposed or working diagnosis
- the proposed treatment and its likely outcome
- the risks associated with this treatment
- the alternative treatments available
- their likely outcomes
- what might happen if no treatment is given.

During this communication you should be invited to ask questions and they should be answered to your satisfaction. You should be asked if you understand what is being proposed and if you wish to go ahead with treatment. If your diagnosis changes down the track, or if a different line of treatment is proposed in future, the informed consent process needs to be commenced again with the new information. Only in this way can both you and the therapist know exactly where you stand in the therapeutic relationship.

Know your rights

As a patient you have the right to revoke your consent at any time and for any reason; this is a safety measure for both parties.

Other sources of information

Once again, doing your homework can pay real rewards. Most clinicians have a presence on the internet. Some have their own home page—check it out. Responsible clinicians tend to be members of professional associations and learned societies. You can look up the web pages of the relevant professional association to check on membership. If not, you can simply telephone the association and ask. You can check with the Australian Health Practitioner Regulation Agency (AHPRA) at www.ahpra.gov.au to confirm that they are registered and in good standing with the board; that is, that there are no complaints, sanctions or notifications against them—which registration authorities sometimes make public. Otherwise, you can do what people have done for centuries—rely on a recommendation. Ask friends or family members who they consult for their back problems. Often the best practitioners develop a following and reputations as being effective therapists. It's not comprehensive but it is a good start.

Our recommendation

Recognise that your health is your responsibility. Although you don't have the technical understanding, you are always in control. It's like having your car repaired. You probably won't have the knowledge and skills of the mechanic or panel beater but that doesn't mean that you give them free reign to do to your car whatever they feel like—without explaining your options and getting your approval. How much more important is it to be a discerning and active participant in the healthcare decisions that you need to make? We believe that you should use the information in this chapter to help you find the right people to help you best manage your back and other health issues. The table below summarises this information. The closer you can arrive at finding therapists with all the positive attributes listed in the table, the sooner you should be enjoying better results.

Not for you?

A particular therapist may not be right for you. Remember, you are under no obligation to have treatment simply because you have had a consultation, diagnosis and discussion. So we advise you seek a second opinion. Unfortunately, the only way to make decisions on whether a therapist is right for you is by trial and error. But don't worry; finding someone who is genuinely able to help you is not difficult, it just means taking control and being discerning.

Expectations

Don't write off a particular therapy unless you have given the therapy a reasonable amount of time to provide results. Ask your practitioner what his or her expectations are regarding your treatment; they may tell you that you will have no significant pain reduction for several weeks. Some conditions may not be able to be fully resolved, so having the expectation that it can be will set you up for disappointment or leave you feeling dissatisfied with your practitioner, neither of which is a positive experience. You should have some level of expectation regarding your treatment, but be careful not to set unrealistic goals. Don't be afraid to try more than one practitioner of a particular therapy—some practitioners are more skilled or experienced than others and they may be able to get you better faster or to a greater degree.

Summary of factors to look for in finding the best practitioner for you

What to look for	Positive attributes	Negative attributes
1. Background		
How did you find this practitioner?	Was referred by a reliable source.	Not referred.
Web check	Web pages appear professional with content that appears reasonable and informative.	Web page is more of a sales pitch than an introduction to the practitioner or services.
Association membership	A member of a professional association or learned society.	Not a member.
2. First consultation		
Knowledge	Appears to be confident in understanding your problem and discussing options that you have. Specialises in problems like yours.	Seems unsure. Appears more interested in trying to convince you of their particular therapeutic approach. Specialises in problems different to yours.
Skill	Physically handled you with confidence. Made you feel secure during physical examination. Made you feel safe during treatment.	You felt awkward when handled. Seemed unsure of what to do next. Made you feel uncomfortable during testing. Made you feel apprehensive during treatment.

Attitude	Greeted you warmly. Was genuinely interested in you. Was a good listener. Gave you their full attention during your consultation. Communicated well with you. Appeared to give you the time you needed on your visit.	You didn't feel welcomed. Treated you like a case rather than an individual. Didn't really listen to you. Allowed distractions during your visit. Communication not satisfying. Appeared to be too rushed.
Informed consent	Explained your diagnosis. Made clear recommendations. Named alternative options. Discussed risks associated with treatment. Allowed you to ask questions. Answered questions to your satisfaction. Asked you to confirm your understanding and acceptance.	Failed to provide a diagnosis, so you had to ask what they thought was going on. Decided on a treatment without discussing it with you. Didn't explain the treatment. Glossed over the risks. You had to seek further information when little or none was offered. Didn't seek your consent.
3. Treatment	Have a trial of treatment. Try the proposed treatment for 1–2 weeks and see if you can find any improvement.	
	You may feel a little better immediately. Your physical exam findings might show early progress. Your ability to do things may improve.	You feel no different after a few treatments. Results of tests such as range of motion don't show any indication of improving. Your disability stays unchanged or gets worse.

6 Back pain and the workplace

Back problems may arise in the workplace, be aggravated by work activities or prevent workers from doing their jobs. While having a back problem can make work very difficult, sometimes it can be impossible to tell whether a person's back problem developed at work, is aggravated by work or is totally unrelated to work.

Sprains and strains of joints and muscles are the most common work injuries. These may involve a single obvious episode of injury or may be caused by a build-up of repetitive injury over time. Other more obvious injuries that arise in the workplace include fractures, crush injuries and bruising. Injury rates can be minimised by adopting a 'safety first' attitude and by using recommended safety equipment. If you do become injured in the workplace, make sure you advise the safety officer as soon as possible regardless of the severity of the injury, and follow all the safety protocols in place at your work site.

Risk factors for developing back pain

Risk factors can be intrinsic (originating within you) or they can be extrinsic (external factors or situations that put you at risk).

Intrinsic risk factors that may increase the chance of you developing back pain include:
- poor muscle tone (especially core/abdominal muscles)
- poor flexibility
- being overweight—the extra weight adds additional compression to the spine

- having previous spinal injuries or past episodes of back pain
- smoking—this could be due to tissue damage in the back caused by smoking or the fact that smokers tend to have unhealthier lifestyles than non-smokers
- pregnancy—the extra weight of carrying a baby can place additional strain on the back
- long-term use of medicine, such as corticosteroids, that is known to weaken bones
- stress—it is thought that stress can cause tension in the muscles of the back, which can result in back pain
- depression—back pain can make people feel depressed, which can result in weight gain leading to more severe pain and worsening depression.

Extrinsic risk factors that may increase the chance of you developing back pain include:

- High work demands:
  - repetitive lifting of heavy objects
  - twisting coupled with bending of the trunk
  - constant, heavy manual work
- whole body vibration
- inability to change or control work patterns
- poor ergonomic design
- stressful work
- poor inter-staff relations
- greater perceived effort at work.

Thankfully, according to the WorkCover Authority of New South Wales, the number of workplace injuries is in decline. This is probably due to better workplace safety strategies that have been adopted over time.

Injury prevention

Back injuries are the largest occupational health and safety problem in Australia. (In New South Wales there is an annual cost of over $500 million in lost production and injury payments.) The prevention of back injuries is complicated but risks can be lowered by following the advice below.

1. Training in safe lifting procedures:
    *   Make sure the weight of the object is within your lifting limit
    *   Get as close as practicable to the object before lifting
    *   Face the object
    *   Use your legs to do the lifting (your back doesn't have to be absolutely straight when you lift)
    *   Use lifting devices or team lifting if the object is heavy
    *   Avoid putting heavy objects on the ground or floor (someone has to lift them up from there)
    *   Don't twist, bend and lift at the same time
    *   See if there is any way to lighten a heavy load before you lift it
    *   Make additional trips rather than overloading yourself
2. Muscle-strengthening exercise programs
3. Flexibility programs
4. Being aware of any weakness that your spine may have (congenital or degenerative) that may predispose you to injury
5. Making sure you are capable of the task—'designing the job to fit the worker'
6. Careful selection of workers

Other than care in lifting, the following strategies can also minimise workplace strain or injury:

*   Maintaining correct posture when sitting and standing
*   Understanding the basic relationship of ergonomics and spinal strain—that is, applied spinal anatomy
*   Being proactive in strategies to avoid back strain.

Posture

Sit, stand and walk like a soldier!
Ever notice a soldier marching or standing at attention with bad posture? Unlikely—they are taught early on in their training to have good posture. We should all strive to emulate them in this capacity.

Good spinal posture is attained not only by standing or sitting up straight, but also by maintaining the arches in your low back and neck, called lordoses. To find the correct position for your low back while standing, place both hands on your low back 3 cm to 4 cm either side of your spine.

Now lean forward; you should feel these muscle contract (become taut). Now lean backward (without bending your knees) arching your back until you feel these muscles go slack. Do these movements several times until you can pinpoint the exact point where the muscles go slack. You have successfully found the neutral position for your low back, which is its ideal position.

The same can be done with your neck. Gently place the fingers of both your hands (palms forward) 2 cm on either side of the back of your neck. Jut your chin forward as far as you can, you should feel the neck muscles underneath your fingers contract and go taut. Now pull your chin backwards until the muscles under your fingers go slack and hold that position. By slowly jutting your chin forward and backward by a few millimeters from this position, you can pinpoint the exact position where your neck muscles relax. You have successfully found the neutral position for your neck, which is your ideal neck posture.

The longer you maintain these postures, the less physical stress or load being placed on your postural muscles. If you can avoid overworking these muscles by maintaining proper posture, you will expend less energy, and be less likely to develop trigger points and adhesions—which means less pain and discomfort and better functioning of your spine.

Forward bending bias

People in modern western society have a propensity towards forward bending of the spine when they sit or stand; some refer to this as **flexion** bias. Desk workers sit for the vast majority of the day. They often commute to work in a seated position, sit at a desk while working until lunch, sit down to have lunch, go back to work for another sitting marathon, go home and sit at the dinner table for dinner, then watch television, work or play on the computer, or read—all of which involve sitting. This is repeated five to seven days per week; no wonder people get sore backs.

Sitting places almost one and a half times as much compression on the spinal discs compared with standing. Slouched sitting places almost three times as much compression on the discs as standing, and also unevenly distributes the load on the disc, with the bulk of the compression force being placed on the **anterior** part of the disc and traction/tension on the back aspect of the disc (refer to the Nachemson chart below). This type of loading causes the jelly-like nucleus to be pushed backwards. Repetition

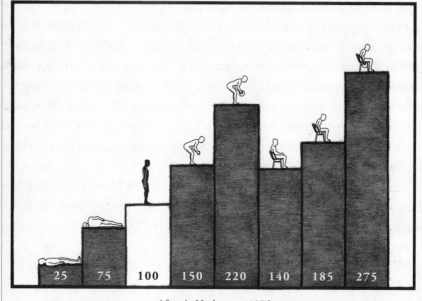

Relative Change in Pressure (or Load) in the Third Lumbar Disc in Various Positions

25   75   100   150   220   140   185   275

After A. Nachemson 1976

of these stresses eventually leads to tearing of the disc fibres, leaving channels (annular fissures) through which the nucleus can ooze. This can lead to a bulging or herniation of the disc and possible nerve compression.

When we sit for a prolonged period of time, several physical changes occur that can lead to low back pain. Postural ligaments that stabilise the spine get stretched. they normally take approximately 30 minutes to stretch to their maximum lengths, after which the body becomes much more reliant on the spinal muscles to maintain upright posture. At this point, the muscles have to do all the work to maintain posture, but they have already worked hard for the past 30 minutes, so as more time passes, the postural muscles begin to fatigue. Then the extensor muscles start to lengthen and the flexor muscles start to shorten. This is why most people begin sitting with good posture, but after approximately 30 minutes must tend to slouch.

As this process is repeated day in and day out, the extensor muscles throughout the spine become locked in a lengthened position, while flexion muscles (like the psoas and rectus abdominis) become locked in a shortened position. Once this occurs, it becomes much more difficult to restore the former posture without therapeutic intervention. At this point soft-tissue treatment is often required to restore proper posture.

How can you combat the forward bending bias? Take more frequent short-duration breaks, called 'micro-breaks', for 1–2 minutes, every 20–30 minutes. Try extending your spine using the seated cat/camel exercise (see the exercise section) for 30–60 seconds. Set your laptop on a counter top or high table so you can work while standing for a while. The body loves variety so switching back and forth from sitting to standing at your workstation is a great way to give you back some variety and rest. Or, try getting some (extra) exercise. Daily movement and exercise in almost any form is helpful in this situation because it gets your joints moving, which lubricates them, increases blood flow to your muscles and assists with circulation, which helps rid your tissues of waste products.

There is no perfect sitting posture

The human body is not designed to maintain a single sitting posture for long periods of time. We've all experienced what it feels like to sit in the same position for too long, we become uncomfortable and fidgety. This is your body telling you to change position! Ideally, you should change sitting position every 10 minutes; this gives certain postural muscles a chance to rest while other muscles are being used. An even better idea is to get out of your chair at least once every 30 minutes in order to unload your spine (see the information on micro-breaks above).

Taking more breaks can actually make you more productive because it is easier to concentrate when your back is not aching.

Good posture can actually make you stronger

You can actually generate more force in a standing posture if you adopt a good upright posture.

Try this little exercise: start your normal standing position and squeeze the hand of a person of your approximate size with a handshake-like grip. Now, we are going to tweak your posture a bit to make you stronger.

185

Stand with your feet slightly wider than hip-width apart and your knees slightly bent. Pull your shoulders down and back by activating your back muscles. Have your neck in a neutral position—not flexed or extended. Make sure you avoid sticking your chin out or tucking it in. Clench your buttocks as firmly as possible like you are trying to crack a nut with your bottom.

Maintain this posture, and then try squeezing the same person's hand with all your might. See if they notice a difference; we bet they will.

Poor posture compresses your spine

Poor spinal posture such as chin jutting, rounded and forward shoulders, and slumping or slouching all lead to over-activation of the erector spinae muscles of the back. The erector spinae muscles are a group of muscles that travel along either side of your spine; they begin at the sacrum and travel all the way up to the base of the skull. When activated, these muscles extend the spine. The term for this posture is 'upper cross syndrome', and it is a pervasive problem in our modern-day, desk-bound work environments. They also cause compression of the intervertebral discs of the spine. Research has shown that if all the erector spinae of an adult contract maximally and simultaneously they can generate enough force to lift a small car off the ground.

When a slouched (upper cross syndrome) posture is maintained for several hours per day, as occurs with most desk-bound workers, the erector spinae muscles are made to work that entire time. Like any skeletal muscle, these ones are not designed to be activated continuously, and they become overworked and fatigue, which causes us to slouch even more. This perpetuates the vicious cycle. The erector spinea muscles become locked in a lengthened (locked long) overstretched position, while muscles in the front of the torso become locked in a shortened position. This throws the front and back myofascial slings out of balance and makes it nearly impossible to maintain good posture. On top of this the erectors begin to develop trigger points (see Chapter 2), which interfere with the function of the muscle and causes them to become sore and weak.

The good news is that you can effectively reverse upper cross syndrome and restore good posture, which will decompress your spine. The first step of the process is to find a good manual practitioner who knows which soft tissues to work on in order to restore proper posture. Your practitioner should also give you some advice on how to minimise your poor posture such as taking micro-breaks or doing the Brügger exercise (see the exercise section) while at work. You should notice some degree of improvement (increased range of motion, better posture, less discomfort, increased muscle strength or endurance) within a matter of weeks. If you don't observe any of these changes after three to four weeks of treatment, you should try another practitioner (see Chapter 5).

A neutral spine is a happy spine

Your spine is happiest in a neutral position—not flexed, extended, rotated, or laterally flexed. In fact all **synovial joints** of the body are most content in a neutral position; this is because a neutral position places the least amount of tension or compression on the joints. Excessive tension or compression of joints is virtually always involved to some degree in painful joints. Being neutral is also the safest position for the spine; this is because it can withstand much greater loads in a neutral position than any other position. Watch world-class Olympic lifters and power lifters—you will see that they always try to maintain a neutral spine. This does not mean that if you maintain a neutral spine you can be super-human; it is simply highlighting the fact that it is the safest, strongest position for the spine.

Ergonomics

In terms of the workplace, this is about 'fitting work to people'. It's the process of designing or arranging workplaces, products and systems so that they fit the people who use them. Think about your job and how well it 'fits' you physically.

Ergonomics considers the physical and mental capabilities of the worker and how he or she interacts with tools, equipment, work methods, tasks and the working environment.

Chairs

Research has demonstrated a correlation between seated work and low back pain. The problem is believed to be due to prolonged and monotonous low-level mechanical load placed on the spine with seated posture.

The most important properties of a chair are the angle of seat pan (the part you sit on), the back rest, the height of the chair and the height of the desk or table you are working at. A seat or a table that is too low will cause you to lean forward, placing you in a bent position, which is bad for your spine. Having your arms supported by arm rests or on a table reduces both spinal muscular activity and disc pressure.

A seat that is angled backwards (negative slope) encourages the lumbar spine to flex, which increases spinal compression. The lumbar spine will flex 35 degrees forward if you sit on a five degrees backward-sloping seat. As the seat angle is increasingly inclined forward, the lumbar spine extends more, which is desired. A five-degree forward slope will result in a 25-degree lumbar flexion, while a 15-degree forward seat slope will reduce the lumbar flexion even further to 15 degrees.

A study evaluated the effects of dynamic (adjustable) office chairs versus fixed (non-adjustable) chairs. They found that dynamic office chairs offer a potential advantage over fixed chairs, but the task performed while seated had a more pronounced effect than that of the chair.

So look for a chair that has adjustability for the seat and back rest angle as well as chair height.

Beds

Beds are very important and you probably spend approximately a third of your life sleeping, so we recommend finding a good one. The trouble is how to discern a good bed from a bad bed. The easiest way to figure it out is literally to sleep on it. Our advice is to buy a bed that you can return or exchange for a different one if you end up not liking it. Go with what is comfortable and what you're used to; if you've always slept soundy in a soft bed don't suddenly decide to get a firm mattress because you read somewhere that firm mattresses are better. Firm mattresses are better for some people, while a soft mattress may be better for others.

Working with back pain—self care

Long-term advice is stay active

Trying to remain active and keep moving should help speed up your recovery. However, acute back pain can be severe and you may need to reduce your activities for a couple of days. Lying in bed or on the couch for longer than this will not help you recover any faster; in fact, it may actually delay your recovery. In the early stage of back pain it is sometimes better to lie rather than sit, but only for short periods of 20–30 minutes at a time.

Gradually increase activities

Keeping the vertebrae and muscles moving is very important, so the sooner you start moving again, the sooner your back is likely to start feeling better. Therefore, it is important to move and stretch regularly, avoid staying in one position (such as sitting at a computer or watching TV). With each day, try to move a little further or faster; slowly build up your level of activity within your normal day-to-day routine. Experiencing some pain when moving is normal, just take it slowly.

Try to get back to work asap

It is highly recommended for people with back pain to return to work fairly quickly. This may mean returning to your work before your pain has completely resolved, and you will probably need to modify your normal work routine until you feel better. This usually means reduced work hours or work activities, and may also mean restrictions on activities such as lifting or prolonged postures. Your healthcare practitioner should discuss this with you and your employer should organise suitable activities when you return to work.

Try to remain positive

Pain can leave you frustrated, sad, worried, angry, tired, or generally in a bad mood. This can make your pain feel even worse. If you feel this way, you are less likely to want to be active, which may slow your recovery. Don't allow the pain to take over. You may find using relaxation techniques such as meditation or yoga, as well as deep-breathing exercises can help you to remain calm and cope with the pain. Try to remember that although the pain may be severe it is likely to be temporary and you should be back to normal within a few days or weeks.

Control the pain

Use pain medication to reduce your pain enough for you to stay active. For most people it is best to start with simple over-the-counter pain-relief medication, such as paracetemol, which does not require a prescription and can be purchased in supermarkets.

Other treatments

Don't just rely on one approach as a strategy to getting better. Research has shown that a combination of treatments, called a multimodal therapy, yields superior results. Consider adding the following:

- manual therapy, such as chiropractic, spinal manipulation, spinal mobilisation and massage
- acupuncture or dry needling
- rehabilitative exercises (such as the ones outlined in the colour section of this book).

Acute injuries

If you have a recent injury, the acronym RICE may help guide you to a better recovery strategy. It is often recommended for an acute injury in the first 24 hours after the injury has occurred:

R: Rest. For the first 24 hours after an acute injury, it is often recommended to reduce activities, as certain activities may exacerbate your injury.

I: Ice therapy. In the first 24 hours after an acute injury, it is recommended to use ice packs to reduce the inflammation process and reduce the severity of the injury. Ice should not be applied directly to the skin and should only be applied for intervals of up to 15 minutes. This can be repeated every one to two hours if the swelling is not reducing.

C: Compression is what this usually stands for. In the first 24 hours after an acute injury it is recommended to compress the area to reduce the inflammation process. However, in terms of the spine, **C = check up**. This means, even if the pain has reduced, it is worthwhile having a spinal therapist review your problem to ensure nothing serious develops.

E: Elevation is the usual meaning. In the first 24 hours after an acute injury it is recommended to elevate the area to reduce the inflammation process. However in the spine **E = exercise**. This means that once the pain has reduced, and a spinal care expert has given you the 'all clear', exercise helps decrease the risk of your problem developing into something serious.

Chronic problems

If you have had your problem more or less continuously for longer than three months, the acronym HEAT is a useful guide:

H = Heat therapy, such as a wheat pack, hot water bottle or heated blanket.

E = Exercise. It is important with chronic injuries to do regular exercise to maintain muscle tone and strength. Even if you experience some pain, it is not necessarily causing more damage.

A = Active. Try to stay as active as possible to avoid joint stiffening or muscle wasting.

T = Treatment. Even if previous treatments haven't given you much benefit, new treatment or treatment approaches may give you some benefit. Within reason, there is nothing to lose by trying something new.

Pharmaceuticals

Non-steroidal anti-inflammatory drugs (**NSAIDs**) are the most frequently prescribed medications worldwide and are widely used for patients with back pain. Also, new anti-inflammatory drugs (COX–2 inhibitors) are widely available and used for patients with back pain.

However, in 65 trials (with a total number of patients 11,237) some positive effects were found in favour of NSAIDs, but at the cost of more side effects:

- There is moderate evidence that NSAIDs are not more effective than paracetamol for acute low back pain, and paracetamol had fewer side effects
- There is moderate evidence that NSAIDs are not more effective than other drugs for acute low-back pain
- There is strong evidence that various types of NSAIDs, including COX–2 anti-inflammatory drugs, are equally effective for acute low back pain.

There does not seem to be a specific type of NSAID that is clearly more effective than others. The COX–2 inhibitor anti-inflammatory drugs showed fewer side effects compared to traditional NSAIDs. However, recent studies have shown that COX–2 inhibitors are associated with increased cardiovascular risks in specific patient populations.

Chronic low back pain

Preventing acute low back injuries from progressing into chronic low back pain syndromes is extremely important. It is estimated that 50 per cent of injured workers who are off work for more than six months will not return to any work, and if they stay out of work for more than 12 months, the return to work rate is almost zero. Work-related back injuries account for a major cause of long-term disability—statistics show that approximately 30 per cent of all workers' compensation claims in Australia are due to acute or chronic low back pain.

The cost for low back pain in Australia was estimated to be $9 billion in 2003, with 5 per cent to 10 per cent of the patients responsible for approximately 75 per cent of the costs (that is, the chronic cases). In addition to medical costs, there are costs related to insurance, disability, employee wage loss, employer replacement and overtime, and legal fees. There is also a substantial burden on injured workers, their families, employers and the workers' compensation systems due to the psychological aspect of chronic low back pain.

Treatment of chronic low back pain usually requires a number of strategies including spinal manipulative therapy (SMT) and multidisciplinary treatment programs. The evidence for SMT clearly shows it can be effective for chronic low back pain. The management of chronic low back pain may include spinal injections, pain medication, and psychological and behavioural therapy. However, few people with chronic low back pain realise they should include spinal manipulative therapy (SMT) as a modality, when the research supports it being included.

Things you can do for yourself to alleviate emotional pain and stress associated with a back problem:

- **Journaling**—just getting your thoughts out of your head and onto paper can take out some of the intensity and help you to see things differently.
- **Self-help reading**—there are some great books and websites to support you to gather tools and techniques to cope more easily. Just be careful to ensure there is an evidence base and professional credentials to back up the material.
- **Looking after your health**—getting enough sleep, exercise and a healthy diet can make a world of difference in how we see and deal

with issues; it can positively influence our body's biochemistry, decrease systemic inflammation, and increase our resilience and brain function to cope.

- **Relaxation strategies**—meditation, yoga, walking, massage or scented baths can help. Enjoy anything that is nurturing and indulgent . . . in moderation!!

Talking it through

Talking to supportive family or friends who you can trust can help—an attentive listener can be a very powerful healing agent. Be careful as often others with the best of intentions stop listening and start telling you what to do, and this rarely helps.

Employee health and wellbeing

Many companies are becoming aware that a healthy and productive workforce is critical for economic success and population health. Illness at the workplace can result in lost productivity, which is now described as absenteeism and presenteeism.

Absenteeism refers to an employee's time away from work due to illness or disability. Presenteeism refers to the decrease in productivity in employees whose health problems have not necessarily led to them being absent from work but have decreased their productivity before or after their absence period. It is defined as being present at work, but limited in some aspects of job performance by a health problem, and it is often a hidden cost for employers. It includes time not spent on job tasks and decreased quality of work (for example, product waste and product defects). Absenteeism and presenteeism are two extremes through which workers may transition back and forth over time.

Preventing back pain

Health promotion in the workplace is defined as preventing, minimising and eliminating health hazards, and maintaining and promoting work ability. Worker health and wellness is maintaining a balance of the physical, mental and social ingredients, as well as maintaining the health habits associated with good physical condition, energy and vitality.

In preventing back pain the responsibility for your health at work ultimately lies with you. Be aware of and follow all workplace-safety directions. Know your limitations—your size, age and gender should be taken into account. Despite their best intentions to create equality at the workplace, many institutions and agencies fail to acknowledge the simple fact that we are not all physically equal. Young men (around 20 years of age) can tolerate more compressive load down their lumbar spines than older men (around 60 years of age) and they can bear a third more load than females of the same age. Compared to older women, studies have shown that young men could tolerate two thirds greater load. By not allowing an unfit 60-year-old woman who weighs 55 kilograms and has osteoporosis to be treated (and protected) differently from a fit 20-year-old male weighing 90 kilograms in terms of tolerating spine load, legislation presents a major barrier to effectively protect workers.

Sleep

The average Australian adult sleeps eight hours per night, and changes position an average of 13 times during this period. Staying awake for 17 straight hours results in a decrease in motor performance equivalent to someone with a blood alcohol-level of 0.05 per cent.

Sleep is important because it is the time the body needs to repair, heal and replenish itself so you feel rested and rejuvenated the next day. If you are getting inadequate sleep, your body does not get enough time to fully repair the wear and tear that has occurred during the day. If this continues, the damage begins to accumulate and the body's physiology begins to exhibit problems. You can increase your sleep quality by exercising, avoiding stimulants like caffeine in the evening, managing stress and improving your diet. In the 1960s, adult Americans were getting an average of 8.5 hours of sleep per night; by 2008 it had dropped to under 7 hours per night. Make getting enough sleep every night a priority in your back care plan. You may benefit in ways you never considered.

My back pain story
Anna Meares

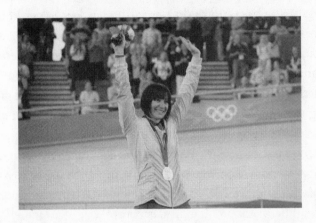

Imagine you are an Olympic cycling gold medallist, and you are seven months away from your second Olympic games in Beijing, where you are one of the favourites to win a gold medal. Disaster strikes; you are flung off your bike travelling 65 kilometres per hour and land on the hard velodrome banking, which fractures your C2 vertebra, dislocates your shoulder, tears multiple tendons and ligaments, and scrapes half the skin off the side of the entire length of your body. Most people would have abandoned any hope of going to the Olympics, but not Anna Meares. Amazingly, Anna got back on a bike within 10 days of the accident, endured daily excruciating rehabilitation sessions and managed to qualify for the Olympics seven months later, where she not only competed, but also won a silver medal.

Anna has struggled with back pain for most of her career, beginning to experience back pain at the age of 22. One morning, after a hard training session the previous night, Anna couldn't get out of bed and immediately knew something was wrong with her back. An MRI of her low back showed that she had damaged three discs of her lumbar spine. Her specialists believed that the damage was due to years of poor lifting posture in the weight room, as well as an imbalance between her core-stability muscles and her back muscles. The first physiotherapist whom she consulted told her it would take at least ten months to recover from her back injury. Anna was not happy with that, so she decided to travel to Adelaide to see the team physiotherapist, who placed Anna on an aggressive back rehabilitation program that focused on retraining her core-stability muscles.

Within three weeks of this new rehab program, Anna was back on the bike, training with the Australian team. Anna began to make changes to her training in an effort to avoid aggravating her low back. This involved changing her sitting position on the bike, using smaller bike gears, which placed less torque on her body, regular stretching and minimising her time in the weight room. At first, Anna would be able to train for a few weeks then her back pain would flare up and she would have to rest and recover for up to a week before she could get back to training. Then after a few more weeks of training her back would flare up again. This cycle continued for the next few years until she and her medical team eventually figured out what activities were beneficial and which ones were detrimental to her back condition. It wasn't until about 2010 that Anna believed she finally had her back problem under control.

Anna continues to suffer from the occasional back problem, but she has learned from her past mistakes and now knows how to treat the cause of her back problems. Nowadays she actively undertakes preventative measures to avert future back problems from occurring, rather than waiting for her back to flare up and then dealing with the problems later. These measures include receiving regular treatment from a physio, chiropractor and a massage therapist to keep her back in good working order.

Anna says avoid being stubborn; she recommends you go out and seek help from those knowledgeable about back pain. She also recommends not being lazy; if your practitioner gives you exercises or stretches—do them. They may seem tedious at times, but they are definitely worthwhile and you will reap the benefits later on.

7 Dos and don'ts

Be careful how far you bend

If you bend forward past 90 degrees of lumbar **flexion**, your back muscles become inactivated. This is known as the 'critical point'. If you bend past the critical point, you no longer have active muscular protection or as much neurological control of the movement of your spine. Therefore, those who work in a bent or stooped position for long durations, such as bricklayers, gardeners or concreters, are at greater risk of injuring the low back region. As a guide, when you bend forward to touch your toes, the critical point is where your fingers tips are past your knees.

The key to working in a bent position is to take frequent short breaks returning your back to an upright neutral position. This avoids fatiguing your back muscles and it decompresses the spine for some time. Another idea is to change tasks several times per day. If you have been doing a job that places you in prolonged bent position, change to a task that requires you to work with an upright posture or even working overhead. This will save your back some anguish and won't cause any loss of productivity.

Don't let 'fear-avoidance behaviour' stop you getting better

People who deal with chronic pain can develop fear-avoidance behaviour. This occurs if you become so fearful of causing yourself pain that you avoid doing many movements or activities you would normally do. This becomes a major problem because the way the body works is, 'if you don't use it, you lose it'. In this scenario you will lose the ability to move or perform certain activities because your body will become deconditioned due to your fear-avoidance behaviour. This in turn could cause you to be unable to generate enough strength or stability to perform various tasks.

In order to better understand fear-avoidance behaviour, we should first define fear. Fear is the emotional reaction to a specific, identifiable and immediate threat, such as a dangerous animal or an injury. Fear can be helpful in circumstances of impending danger as it instigates the fight or flight response, which can save us from danger. Fear and anxiety are terms that are commonly used interchangeably when it comes to pain. However, anxiety is when we concern ourselves with what might happen in the future, and these 'what if' situations do not necessarily happen. An important component of anxiety is hyper-vigilance, which is when an individual continually scans their environment in order to detect any potential sources of threat. Both fear-avoidance behaviour and hyper-vigilance can be counterproductive in the long term, eventually promoting disability and disuse.

If you are concerned that you could be suffering from fear-avoidance behaviour or hyper-vigilance, you need to talk to your practitioner about your fears and what it is that has you anxious about receiving treatment. A good practitioner will be empathetic to your fears and, instead of making adjustments, they could just talk to you about treatment options or make a plan with you about what you will do each session. Treatment does not have to be a quick process; if you need to take it slowly, just advise your practitioner.

Get your bone density checked

Bone density in females is set by 18 years of age; in males it's set at 22 years. From then on, your bone density slowly declines as you age. The normal decline after 35 years of age is 1 per cent per year for cortical bone (the hard, outer shell of bones), and 2 per cent per year for cancellous bone (the inner, spongy bone) per year. At menopause, the rate of bone loss increases tenfold; certain areas such as the lumbar spine can increase to as much as 20-fold or 6 per cent per year.

Researchers have come up with a formula for calculating the percentage of bone loss per year based on your age. For a 60-year-old woman the average bone density loss is 2 per cent per year. Studies repeatedly demonstrated that resistance training is one of the most effective ways to maintain your bone density. That's why astronauts work out on the space station or shuttle, to counter the bone density loss from zero gravity.

There are several simple non-invasive methods of testing bone density. The current gold standard is dual energy X-ray absorptiometry (DEXA). Another commonly performed test is an ultrasound of the heel. Be sure to get your bone density tested if you are over 50 years old; men should get it done as well. Women over 60 years old should have their bone density checked every three years.

The leg press machine can damage your low back

The leg press machine is dangerous for low backs. The reason is that it can exert tremendous compression forces on the lumbar spine. Leg press machines cause the pelvis to rotate away from the back rest as your knees come down toward your chest. This leads to compression (pinching) of the front of the lumbar discs, and distraction (stretching) of the **posterior** aspect of the disc. Add to that a very heavy load (many people use these machines to stack on the weight plates to show off) and you have the perfect recipe to destroy your lumbar discs. Experts who specialise in low back biomechanics and pain research are trying to get these machines banned from gyms because of their damaging effects on the low back.

Furthermore, leg press is not a functional movement. Think about it: how often do you get into a 45-degree inclined seated position just a few centimetres off the floor and push a heavy load up a ramp? For most people the answer is never. So, why do an exercise in a position you never get into? If you want to work your legs, stick with the basics: squats, lunges, deadlifts and step-ups. When performed properly, these exercises will work all the big muscle groups of the lower body and are safe for most people when done properly.

Work on increasing core stabiliby endurance, not strength

Research has shown that decreased core-stability muscle endurance is predictive of low back pain. You can increase your core-stability endurance by learning spine-sparing core-stability exercises (refer to exercise section in this book). They are not difficult to do, but need to be done properly. Even if you learn them from this book, it is a worthwhile process to consult a professional who can observe your technique and correct you if you are doing it improperly. If done properly, these exercises improve the endurance of the core stabilisers and can make a huge difference in how your back feels and functions. So, work on increasing your core-stability endurance, not strength; it will make a big difference to your back in the future.

Avoid lifting in the first hour after waking

Because the intervertebral discs are thicker in the morning, the pressure inside the disc is greater, which for those with damaged or unhealthy discs leads to greater discomfort or pain or both. One hour after rising, the discs have lost 90 per cent of the thickness they gained overnight, and back pain sufferers gain some relief.

This information is useful if you plan on working out first thing in the morning, or if your job requires heavy or repetitive lifting soon after waking. If this is the case for you, there is a simple solution; simply wake up at least an hour before you begin any manual labour or exercise. It will save your discs a lot of unnecessary stress and strain, and can prevent unnecessary low back pain.

Once a disc is damaged it will remain permanently altered; however, this does not necessarily imply that the disc will be painful forever. Changing your activities and behaviours to avoid or diminish further damaging effects on the spine can significantly improve your back pain symptoms, and potentially prevent future problems.

Power walking is good for bad backs

When you walk briskly, your arms swing to and fro—further than when walking at a slow pace. Greater arm swinging causes greater activation of you abdominal oblique muscles. This in turn causes a stiffening of your core that stabilises your spine better. The end result—your back hurts less! So, if you have back troubles and are capable of walking, try walking at a brisk pace to further activate your core-stability muscles and ease your back pain.

If you have a bad back, don't do sit-ups

Standard sit-ups or crunches, where you lay on your back with your knees bent to 90 degrees and curl up as far as you can, place a lot of stress on the spine, especially the spinal discs. A normal sit-up (as described above) places 3200 N of force on the spine. The National Institute for Occupational Safety and Health suggests a limit for workplace low back forces of 3000 N. Based on these guidelines, if you do a single sit-up, you are exceeding your spine's safe range. Yet very often people with back problems are wrongly advised to do sit-ups to try to get better. Unfortunately, they are causing even greater damage to their spines in doing so, and may perpetuate or aggravate their low back pain until they stop.

There are safe ways to work your core muscles without doing sit-ups or other exercises that place large forces on the spine. They are called 'spine-sparing exercises'. Spine-sparing core-stability exercises have been clinically tested to ensure that they do not exceed the force limits for the spine. Professor Stuart McGill has developed a set of these exercises that work the core muscles without stressing or compressing the spine. McGill calls them 'the Big 3', and each exercise focuses on one of the three areas of the torso: the **anterior**, **posterior** and **lateral** sides (these exercises are described in detail in the colour section). By focusing on each of these areas, the four quadrants of the core are covered and progressive improvements can be attained.

Try walking with a backpack for low back pain

Wearing a well-supported backpack loaded with 10 kilograms decreases the compressive load on the spine. Most people tend to slouch when they walk; those with low back issues tend to exaggerate this posture even more. A weighted backpack has the positive effect of pulling the spine into a more upright posture. By placing the spine in a more natural lordotic posture, the erector spinae muscles are effectively turned off. This decreases the compressive forces acting on the spine and unloads the spine. Try it and see how you go.

Learn to belly breathe

Most people breathe through the chest and not with the belly. When you belly breathe you activate your diaphragm, which is your main and most powerful respiratory muscle and the only respiratory muscle that does not fatigue. When you breathe in (inspiration) your belly should naturally bulge outward, because your diaphragm lies in a horizontal plane across your torso. When you breathe in, the diaphragm moves down, compressing the organs in the torso. This in turn pushes out against the abdominal walls and makes the belly bulge outward. Many relaxation and meditation therapies take advantage of the benefits of belly breathing to relax the body and calm the mind.

Some people actually do the exact opposite and the belly goes inward during inspiration. This is called 'reciprocal or paradoxical breathing'. Reciprocal breathing is an unwanted respiratory pattern, as it restricts the amount of oxygen you take in with every breath, causing you to take shorter and more frequent breaths. Furthermore, it makes the 'secondary respiration muscles' such as those in your neck activate to a greater degree, which in turn makes them tighter and prone to develop trigger points.

Belly breathing is also more energy efficient; we expend less energy when belly breathing because we use fewer muscles and we need to take fewer breaths to take in the same amount of oxygen. There are many benefits to belly breathing and virtually no negative effects, so what are you waiting for? Start belly breathing!

Breathing properly can be a very important component of core-stability training and your recovery. Your diaphragm is your main and strongest respiratory muscle. During normal breathing the diaphragm will contract and relax, which is desired. If you hold your breath during an exercise, your body will not be able to transport oxygen to your muscles and your muscles will enter anaerobic (without oxygen) metabolism. Most individuals have an anaerobic capacity of only about 60 seconds. If the exercise you are performing takes longer than 60 seconds to complete, you are going to run into a major road block. Professor McGill has demonstrated that taking short interval breaks while performing core-stability exercises allows muscles to take in some oxygen, which in turn permits greater muscle force production and less fatigue.

Avoid sitting on your wallet

A common practice among males is to place their wallet in their back pocket. This is fine when you are standing or walking; however, it has negative effects when you sit on your wallet. There is even a term for what it causes: 'wallet sciatica'. Here are a few reasons sitting on your wallet is not good for you.

First, the wallet props up your pelvis on the side of the wallet, messing up your pelvic alignment. The wallet pushes the pelvis on the wallet side up and forward compared to the other side. This is an undesirable effect, as it is biomechanically inefficient to have the pelvis misaligned, and it can cause back pain such as sacroiliac joint dysfunction. Secondly, the wallet digs into several important muscles in your buttocks (gluteus maximus/ medius/minimus, piriforimis, gemelli and obturator muscles) and can lead to the formation of trigger points, adhesions and scar tissue. Adhesions in some of these muscles can cause nerve entrapment of the sciatic nerve, which can lead to neurological symptoms (sciatica) in the lower limb such as pain, numbness, pins and needles or weakness. Once these adhesions form, they are difficult to get rid of and you will most likely require some form of manual therapy in order to resolve the problem.

These situations can be avoided by simply not sitting on your wallet.

Get worked on, even when you feel good

We recommend getting worked on even when you're feeling good. Most patients seek treatment only when they have a specific complaint or injury. However, a small percentage of patients will present with no major complaint, just a desire to be 'checked up'. The great thing about these patients is that the clinician is not forced to focus on an injured area, and is free to look for functional problems throughout the body.

Out of 100 people, 99 will have some biomechanical dysfunction somewhere in the body, so why not fix them before they become a problem and while they are pain free? For one, it is a great way to prevent injuries from occurring and, secondly, it is often far less painful to be worked on because the area is not inflamed. We recommend you get worked on at least once a month, even if you feel good. Good practitioners will find problems you didn't even know you had, which can prevent future serious problems from arising.

Everything in moderation

This old adage rings true for low backs. One study demonstrated that, overall, people with sedentary (desk-bound) jobs had more low back problems then labourers. The reason is because labourers move and use their muscles. Sedentary workers tend not to move or use their back and core-stability muscles. If you don't use it, you lose it! Those muscles atrophy (shrink) and become less functionally capable of doing their respective jobs. By contrast, labourers often overload or over-use their backs, which can also cause damage. The moral of the stories is that your back needs a happy medium; not too much physical work and not too much sedentary work.

If seeing multiple practitioners, take the team approach

The reasons you don't want to see multiple health practitioners in isolation are simple. First, it makes it impossible for the practitioners to coordinate a treatment plan. Second, it can lead to confusion and discrepancies in terms of scheduling, particularly if you have appointments at different locations. Also, it can be expensive. We suggest starting with one practitioner and sticking with them for a trial period of one month. Ask the practitioner if they believe they can completely resolve the problem or, if it can't be resolved, what kind of symptomatic benefits you should expect to see with treatment.

If after a one-month trial period you have not had any improvements, it is time to move on. Try to find a practitioner who has a planned treatment program for you, and is not just flying by the seat of their pants. Also avoid practitioners who do exactly the same treatment on every patient; odds are, they'll treat you the same way. (See our advice on how to choose a good practitioner for your back pain in Chapter 5.)

However, keep in mind that sometimes it is necessary to consult more than one practitioner if different therapy approaches are required simultaneously. For instance, you may need acupuncture, spinal manipulation and medication. It is important that all the practitioners involved in your management are aware of each other's involvement and work in a team approach.

Always find out your diagnosis

At the end of your examination be sure to ask your practitioner for a diagnosis or differential diagnosis. If the diagnosis is too difficult for you to remember, have your practitioner write it down for you and keep it in a safe place where you won't lose it. If you decide to consult other practitioners, any previous diagnoses are valuable information. If your previous treatment was unable to improve your condition, it is likely that the diagnosis was incorrect or the treatment was inappropriate or ineffectively applied. This information helps practitioners come up with a more precise diagnosis or a better treatment approach, which leads to better results for you.

Don't sleep on your stomach

Sleeping on your stomach (prone) is bad for you. Why? It restricts your breathing. When we breathe, our ribs move upward and outward to allow our lungs to fill with air. If the rib movement is restricted, less air can be taken in by the lungs. Sleeping prone is also bad for your neck. Generally, in order to breathe while lying prone, you have to rotate the head at least 45 degrees. This causes the muscles on one side of your neck to lengthen and the other side to shorten. After several hours of this maintained posture, certain muscles will develop trigger points, which can cause neck pain and headaches.

Alleviating back pain while you sleep

Sleep with a pillow between your knees when you sleep on your side or a pillow under your knees if you sleep on your back.

If you prefer sleeping on your side, try to alternate sides (unless one side sets off your back pain) or try sleeping on your back occasionally.

Purchasing a new mattress can often make a big difference in how back pain sufferers feel when they sleep, because the material in beds breaks down with use and generally only lasts about eight years. Some people do better with a harder mattress and others with a softer mattress. The best advice is to purchase a mattress from a store that will allow you to change the mattress (at no extra cost) if it is not to your liking.

Avoid drinking a lot of fluid just before bed—the more you drink, the more likely you will have to get up in the middle of the night to go to the toilet. This is particularly true for seniors.

If lying on your stomach is the only position you can sleep in, try placing a pillow beneath your abdomen and avoid using a pillow for your head.

Pack your running shoes

These days businesspeople wear aesthetically pleasing but often uncomfortable footwear, all in the name of fashion. In the business world many men wear rigid loafers and women wear high-heeled shoes, which can cause lower limb repetitive strain injuries over time. If you walk longer than five minutes, you should put on a pair of walking or running shoes. A good idea is to pack your runners in a bag and bring them with you to work. Pull them on for that long walk to and from the office, and then simply swap them for your more fashionable shoes once you get to work. Walking and running shoes are far more comfortable because they are designed to bend where your foot naturally wants to flex, have more built-in cushioning to absorb shock, are often lighter and often provide much better foot support.

Move it or lose it!

The majority of the body's joints are what are called **synovial joints**. These are freely movable joints in which adjacent bony surfaces are covered by cartilage and connected by a fibrous capsule lined with a synovial membrane. The synovial membrane makes synovial fluid, which lubricates the joint. A problem with synovial joints is that in order to stay well-lubricated, movement is required. The full range of movement can sometimes be difficult to attain with normal activities of daily living. Without proper lubrication, the cartilage begins to degenerate. As cartilage degeneration progresses, other dysfunctions begin to show up such as reduced range of movement, painful movement and crepitus (the creaking sound that worn joints make). This progression can be slowed or avoided if we simply move our joints. This is where exercises such as yoga, pilates, tai chi and dance are helpful because they get us to move in ways that are not common in our everyday lives. Other methods of achieving these movements are by doing active mobilisations (see the exercise section).

Micro-breaks

These are very short rests that you take while at work—generally 30–120 seconds but taken frequently throughout the workday. Many patients frown when told they need to take more breaks; they often say 'I'm too busy' or 'I forget to do it'. These two excuses can be easily circumvented. With micro-breaks the ideal frequency is approximately one micro-break every 20–30 minutes. If you work an eight-hour workday, that would be a minimum of 16 breaks (not factoring in a lunch or tea break). So, if you took 16 micro-breaks at 60 seconds each you have a total of 16 minutes breaking over an eight-hour period. Honestly, if you can't fit in 16 minutes worth of time in an eight-hour workday you should have better time management.

Now on to the next excuse: 'I simply forget to take a break'. There are a number of ways to remind yourself to take a break. It is recommended that office workers take a break approximately every 20–30 minutes. One method is to set a timer on the other side of the room from where you sit, which forces you to get up and walk over to the timer to turn it off. If you don't have a timer, you can download a program onto your computer that has a pop-up that prompts you to take a break. You can even set a reminder on your smartphone (on vibrate so you don't disturb your co-workers) to notify you to take a break. After a while you will develop a habit of taking regular micro-breaks and it won't seem like such as task. The benefits are worth it.

If it hurts, don't do it!

New patients inevitably ask the same question at the end of the first treatment: 'What activities/stretches/exercises should I do and which should

I avoid?' A simple rule is, 'If it hurts, don't do it!' Patients who present with knee pain often go on to explain that the knee hurts when they go for a run. However, despite this, they continue to run because they think that they should simply toughen up and push through the pain barrier. That doesn't sound like a logical way to get that knee to feel any better. Every time patients like this go for a run they are irritating some structure in their body, causing their knees to hurt. The 'hurt' structure then sends signals up to the brain that are interpreted as pain. The human body is constantly sending and receiving signals via the nervous system. These signals let us know how our body is functioning in real-time. If a movement hurts, that usually means that something may be dysfunctional. The goal is to figure out what is dysfunctional, and why, and then treat the cause.

There are exceptions to this rule. Some therapies, such as yoga and McKenzie treatment, involve some degree of pain, but not hurt. If you are concerned that the activities are causing harm, you should consult with an experienced, qualified person.

Try going barefoot

Barefoot walking is good for us, on the right surfaces. Most of us wear some form of footwear every day. Certain shoes can limit the flexibility and mobility of the foot. People walked barefoot for thousands of years when concrete pathways and asphalt roads did not exist. However, nowadays most urban areas we walk on are hard, perfectly flat surfaces. Concrete and asphalt are so hard and dense that if we walked barefoot on them all the time we would all end up with stress fractures in our lower limbs. We can, however, go places where walking barefoot is ideal. Walking on soft sand and grass are great surfaces to walk on barefoot.

The benefits of walking barefoot are it stimulates the nerves in our feet, which in turn helps with balance, it stimulates blood flow, and it gets multiple joints in the feet moving, providing vital lubrication to these joints.

Train smarter, not harder!

The old adage 'no pain, no gain' is seldom viable and often foolishly followed.

Pain should not be your goal when exercising. Sometimes we hear patients say, 'I had an awesome workout—I could hardly walk the next day.' That should not be your goal. The aim when exercising is to improve athletic attributes such as speed, endurance, strength, power, stability and dexterity. So why not train the attributes that will benefit you most in your chosen sport? If you are a marathon runner, you would most likely want to work on endurance. You would probably not want to focus on strengthening your biceps as it will not enhance your endurance or improve your marathon time. Try making a list of all the athletic attributes that are most beneficial in your sport of choice. If you are not sure what they are, do some research to find out. Once you know which attributes you want to train, find out the most appropriate training regimen to maximise these attributes. Many recreational athletes make the error of thinking that the best way to train for their sport is to train like the professionals do. They forget that professionals are highly skilled in their sport, which results in fewer errors of performance and a significantly decreased likelihood of injury. If an average person were to try to train like a professional—without the years of experience, coaching, hand–eye coordination, core stability, speed, agility and dexterity—the results could prove disastrous. Start by finding out what the most appropriate training regimen for you in your selected sport would be at your current physical status, and then build from there.

Too much bed rest can make your back worse

Studies on prolonged bed rest demonstrate that it can make your back pain worse. Research has shown that bed rest (compared with advice to stay active) has harmful effects on back pain patients. This is because prolonged bed rest reduces blood supply to certain areas and thus slows healing and recovery. When you lie horizontal the compression gravity normally exerts on your spine is removed, and the disc begins to soak up water like a sponge. The longer the bed rest, the more the intervertebral discs inflate with water. What eventually occurs is that once the discs have soaked up as much water as they can, the pressure inside the disc, termed 'intradiscal pressure', is so great that it causes low back pain. Add this to the fact that those often prescribed bed rest are already in moderate to severe pain and you have a recipe for disaster. Current research states that bed rest should be used for a maximum of three days. Gradual resumption of activity is what is best. Pain is not a good guide because even appropriate activities can be uncomfortable for back pain sufferers. Allowing pain to be a guide leads to activity avoidance and deconditioning, which is not what you want.

Always check your medications for side effects

All drugs have the potential to cause serious side effects. These side effects can happen when you start a new medication, decrease or increase dosage of a medication or stop using a medication. That is why it is so important to always read the label of your medication. If the label is missing or you want more information, you can get it from a pharmacist or your doctor. You can also look it up on the internet; however, be sure to only use reliable sites such as the drug manufacturer or a government health agency. Medication side effects can often be the cause of many complaints that health practitioners see in practice. Fortunately it is usually an easy problem to fix.

The following changes require you to work with your physician and have their advice before proceeding: trying a different medication, or making lifestyle and health changes in order to try to reduce or get off the medication. Always mention to any health practitioner you are consulting what medications you are currently taking or have recently stopped taking. Even if they don't ask—some practitioners may forget to ask—volunteer it freely so it can't be missed.

Keep a copy of your medical history

Always keep an up-to-date copy of your medical history. This information can easily be printed out by your doctor or summarised onto a couple of sheets of paper. Simply call your general practitioner's office and request a printed copy of your medical history and up-to-date list of medications, including dosages. Once you have these sheets, make a few copies and keep a copy in a safe place. Also having a copy in your wallet or handbag when you consult a new health practitioner is a great idea. You can help your parents or grandparents to obtain their history as well. We're sure they'll appreciate the effort.

Good technique reduces injury

If you were a sporty child, think back to your school days when you played sport—did you work on technique? Of course you did; that was the point of going to training and practice sessions. Even professional athletes continue to work on their technique. They work on technique for two primary reasons: firstly, to improve athletic performance and, secondly, to avoid and prevent injury.

'Weekend Warriors' is a term commonly used to describe non-professional athletic people. These are athletes who compete in sports that usually take place over the weekend. Often these athletes fail to train or practise adequately during the week due to time constraints. This leads to a lack of physical fitness, which in turn leads to a decreased capacity to execute specific athletic movements and also leads to poor technique. An easy solution is to practise! Even if it's just for half an hour twice a week. The best option is to go to a sports coach. This will serve two purposes: improve technique and enhance physical fitness, both of which will lead to enhanced athletic performance and decrease the risk of injury.

Drink more water

Water makes up approximately two-thirds of the human body and is essential for life, yet most people walk around in a mild state of dehydration every day. A simple way to see if you are dehydrated is to examine the colour of your urine. Urine should be clear or transparent; if it is yellow, you are dehydrated (note that if you are taking vitamins, these can alter the colour of your urine). The darker the yellow, the more dehydrated you are. Water plays a part in almost all vital bodily functions. Adequate fluid intake helps with body temperature regulation and maintains adequate blood volume. The average person loses 250 millilitres of water per day just from breathing! Maintaining proper hydration not only is necessary for life but also improves fitness and reduces risks of problems or injury due to fluid loss. You can calculate how much water you lose while exercising by first weighing yourself before exercising and then weighing yourself after exercising. One kilogram of weight loss equals one litre of water; that is, one gram per millilitre.

Learn eccentric exercises

An eccentric contraction is when a muscle is lengthened while contracting under a load. Studies have demonstrated that these are some of the most effective exercises available for treating and preventing tendon problems. Most exercises that people perform involve concentric contractions, which is when a contracted muscle shortens under load. One of the reasons that eccentric exercises work so well is that it significantly reduces the forces placed on a muscle or tendon, thus providing a safer exercise, but with all the same benefits of the concentric exercise. A squat is a good example of an exercise that involves eccentric muscle activity.

Learn self-mobilisations

Mobilisations are techniques used to decrease pain and increase joint range of motion. Mobilisations are not stretches; stretches act on muscles, **fascia** and tendons. Mobilisations act on joints. Mobilisations can be done either actively (you do it to yourself) or passively (the movement is done to you by someone else). Self-mobilisations are done actively and may be slightly uncomfortable, but they should not reproduce pain. If mobilisation of your spine causes pain, you are either moving past your tolerable range of motion or your spine is too injured or dysfunctional to move into that range. If you experience pain during the mobilisation near the end of your range of motion, try using a shorter range of motion to begin with. This is called the pain-free range of motion, and it is helpful when first starting mobilisations or when pain is particularly severe. An example of a good spinal self-mobilisation is the cat/camel exercise (see colour section).

Conclusion

We would like to congratulate you for getting through this book, and we hope you will benefit from the insight and information we have provided. Unfortunately, back pain continues to have an enormous social and economic burden throughout the world. This does not need to be the case; with the advent of evidence-based management for back pain, this burden can be significantly reduced. We must erase the fear and confusion regarding back pain. Study after study demonstrates that chronic back pain is not a life sentence; conversely, people tend to improve with time and proper care. Acute back pain frequently has a good prognosis and is quickly resolved, despite having a common recurrence rate. Researchers and practitioners are continually working on new treatments and new technologies to help solve the conundrum of back pain. More research on back pain needs to be carried out and, although we may never fully understand back pain and its causes, we should never stop searching for answers.

We hope that you will periodically refer back to certain chapters of this book or even re-read it from time to time, as some of the concepts and recommendations are easily forgotten. Although the science of back pain will continue to progress in the future, many basic principles that we have outlined in this book will remain the same. If you have a friend or family member who suffers from back pain, don't be afraid to share the insight you have gained from this book; you may be able to save them from the debilitating effects of back pain. Better yet, lend them your copy or purchase a copy for them so they too can benefit from the information within.

We think that the colour exercises section in this book can make a dramatic contribution to getting your back better and helping you stay well. Take the book to your therapist and ask their advice on which exercises are best for you.

We suggest that you carefully consider the information that we have provided in this book. When used properly and in the appropriate circumstances, most people can achieve great results. We also trust this book has cleared up some commonly held misconceptions about back pain, its diagnosis and treatment.

We expect that this book has helped you and many other back pain sufferers. If we are able to help just one person from the writing of this book, it will have been worth the effort. Back pain, particularly chronic back pain, can be one of the hardest things for some to overcome in life. It may even be debilitating but do not be dissuaded or discouraged. It can take a long time to overcome, but where there is a will, there is a way.

We have plans to develop a smartphone app based on this book to help you with your exercises and to monitor your progress. If you liked our book or would like to leave a comment, please visit our website: www.treatthecause.com.au. It contains information on back pain, links to other great sites on back pain and a Q & A section.

Glossary

abduction movement of a limb away from the midline of the body

absolute contraindication a situation that absolutely forbids the use of a particular treatment

active trigger point a tender spot in a muscle that refers pain in a particular pattern and can restrict movement

adduction movement of a limb toward the midline of the body

analgesia lack of sensation

anatomical position the reference point to describe the position of one body part relative to another. It involves standing, facing forwards with the palms facing forwards

antalgia a posture adopted to avoid or minimise pain

anterior towards the front

cavitation the 'pop' or 'crack' sound that is made when a joint is manipulated

collagen the most abundant protein in mammals; a major component of *fascia*, giving it strength and flexibility

contraindication a factor that prohibits the administration of a drug or the performance of an act or procedure in the care of a specific patient

extension the process of straightening, moving away from *flexion* or the state of being straight

fascia a tissue that covers and binds body tissues; it is an uninterrupted, three-dimensional web of tissue that extends from head to toe

fibroblast a connective-tissue cell that secretes collagen from which connective tissue forms

fibrosis fibrous degeneration; abnormal increased deposition of fibrous tissue

flexion the process of bending or the state of being bent

fracture a broken bone; there are various sub-classes of fractures—for example, compound, stress, compression

hyperreflexia overactivity of physiological reflexes

hypoxia a situation where insufficient oxygen reaches the tissues

indication a reason to prescribe a medication or perform a treatment

inferior anatomically more distant from the head—for example, the low back is inferior to the thorax

joint capsule the envelope which borders a *synovial joint*

kyphosis a *posterior* convex curvature of the spine; it occurs naturally in the thoracic spine and the sacrum/coccyx complex

latent trigger point muscle dysfunction that restricts range of motion in the affected muscle but does not cause local or referred pain

lateral furthest from the middle of the body

lateral flexion to bend to the side, or to be side-bent

lordosis concave curve of the back of the spine; it occurs naturally in the cervical and lumbar spine

mechanoreceptors cells specialising in sensing movement

medial nearer the middle of the body

meniscus/menisci a cartilage disc that acts as a cushion between the ends of bones that meet in a joint

myofascia connective surrounding and joining muscle and *fascia*

NSAIDs non-steroidal anti-inflammatory drugs

osteophyte a degenerative bony spur formation commonly arising from a vertebral body or facet joint

periosteum a dense membrane composed of fibrous connective tissue that closely wraps (invests) all bone

posterior towards the rear—for example, the brain is posterior to the eyes

radiculopathy nerve pain, sensory impairment, weakness or diminished deep tendon reflexes in a nerve root distribution

recumbent lying down

referred pain pain perceived at a location other than the site of the painful stimulus

relative contraindication a situation that may forbid the use of a particular treatment

rotation circular movement around a central axis, such as twisting the spine

scoliosis an abnormal *lateral* curvature of the spine

spinal stenosis narrowing of the spinal canal that may result in bony constriction of the cauda equina and the emerging nerve roots

synovial joint the most common type of joint in the body—for example, the knee

tendinosis degenerative condition of a tendon

TheraBand an exercise aid composed of elastic sheeting that provides resistance when stretched; available in different thicknesses for variable resistance

viscera organs or organ systems of the human body

VMO vastus medialis obliqus muscle

References

The following sources were used in the compilation of this book. Our search of the literature found the following scientific articles, which would be useful for anyone wishing to follow up on specific areas of enquiry. We have divided the references into categories, although there is substantial overlap of topics between these sources. If you would like to find highly detailed information on back pain topics, the sources below are an excellent place to start.

In many cases the whole papers are available on the web; otherwise, the abstracts can be accessed. The abstracts from these papers can be found using either a PubMed search or a Google Scholar search. Respectively, those search page addresses are www.ncbi.nlm.nih.gov/pubmed/ and http://scholar.google.com.au/.

Scientific journal articles

Acute back pain
Schroth WS, Schectman JM, Elinsky EG, et al. 'Utilization of medical services for the treatment of acute low back pain: conformance with clinical guidelines'. *J Gen Intern Med* 1992, 7:486–91

Chronic low back
Deyo RA, Mirza SK, Turner JA, et al. 'Overtreating chronic back pain: Time to back off?'. *J Am Board Fam Med.* 2009, 22:62–68

Cost of back pain
Adams MA, McNally DS, Wagstaff J, et al. 'Abnormal stress concentrations in lumbar intervertebral discs following damage to the vertebral bodies: a cause of disc failure?'. *Eur Spine J.* 1993, 1:214–221
AIHW 2012. 'Australia's health 2012'. *Australia's health* no. 13. Cat. no. AUS 156. Canberra: AIHW.

Becker A, Held H, Redaelli M, Strauch K, Chenot JF, Leonhardt C, et al. 'Low back pain in primary care: costs of care and prediction of future health care utilization'. *Spine.* 2010 Aug, 35(18):1714–20. PubMed PMID: MEDLINE:21374895.

Crownfield P. 'Back pain is #1 cause of disability worldwide—Global Burden of Disease 2010 highlights the pressing need to prevent, treat spinal and musculoskeletal disorders'. *Dynamic Chiropractic.* 2013, 31(4).

Deyo RA, Cherkin D, Conrad D, Volinn E. 'Cost, controversy, crisis: low back pain and the health of the public'. *Annual review of public health.* 1991, 12:141–56

Furlan AD, Yazdi F, Tsertsvadze A, et. al. 'A systematic review and meta-analysis of efficacy, cost-effectiveness, and safety of selected complementary and alternative medicine for neck and low-back pain'. *Evid Based Comp Alt Med.* 2012, 2012:953139.

Mehra M, Hill K, Nicholl D, Schadrack J. 'The burden of chronic low back pain with and without a neuropathic component: a health-care resource use and cost analysis' *Journal of medical economics.* 2012 Dec, 15(2):245–52. PubMed PMID: MEDLINE:22136441.

Swedlow A, Johnson G, Smithline N, et al. 'Increased costs and rates of use in the California workers' compensation system as a result of self-referral by physicians'. *N Engl J Med.* 1992, 327:1502–6.

Vos T et al. 'Years lived with disability (YLDs) for 1160 sequelae of 289 diseases and injuries 1990—2010: a systematic analysis for the Global Burden of Disease Study 2010'. *The Lancet,* Volume 380, Issue 9859, Pages 2163–2196, 15 December 2012

Walker BF, Muller R, Grant WD. 'Low back pain in Australian adults: the economic burden'. *Asia-Pacific journal of public health* / Asia-Pacific Academic Consortium for Public Health. 2003, 15(2):79–87. PubMed PMID: MEDLINE:15038680.

Walker BF, Muller R, Grant WD. 'Low back pain in Australian adults: health provider utilization and care seeking'. *Journal of manipulative and physiological therapeutics.* 2004, 27(5):327–35. PubMed PMID: MEDLINE:15195040.

Disc problems

Adams M & Roughley P. 'What is intervertebral disc degeneration, and what causes it?' *Spine.* 2006, 31(18):2151–2161.

Aprill C, Bogduk N. 'High-intensity zone: a diagnostic sign of painful lumbar disc on magnetic resonance imaging'. *The British Journal of Radiology.* 1992, 65 (773):361–369

Beggs I, Addison J. 'Posterior vertebral rim fractures'. *Br J Radiol.* 1998, 71:567–572

References

Brinckmann P, Frobin W, Hierholzer E, et al. 'Deformation of the vertebral end-plate under axial loading of the spine'. *Spine.* 1983, 8:851–856

Fardon D, & Milette P. 'Nomenclature and classification of lumbar disc pathology: Recommendations of the Combined Task Forces of the North American spine Society, American Society of Spine Radiology, and American Society of Neuroradiology'. *Spine.* 2001, 26(5):93–113

Hansson TH, Keller TS, Spengler DM. 'Mechanical behaviour of the human lumbar spine. II. Fatigue strength during dynamic compressive loading'. *J Orthop Res.* 1987, 5:479–487

Humzah MD, and Soames RW. 'Human intervertebral disc: structure and function'. *Anat Rec.* 1988, 220:337–356

Kang CH. 'Treatment of internal disc derangement by posterior lumbar interbody fusion and posterior instrumentation'. *State of the art for minimally invasive spine surgery.* 2005, 87–97

Moneta GB, Videman T, Kaivanto K, et al. 'Reported pain during lumbar discography as a function of anular ruptures and disc degeneration. A re-analysis of 833 discograms'. *Spine.* 1994, 17:1968–1974

Moore RJ, Vernon-Roberts B, Fraser RD. 'The origin and fate of herniated lumbar intervertebral disc tissue'. *Spine.* 1996, 21:2149–2155

Moore RJ. 'The vertebral end-plate: disc degeneration, disc regeneration'. *Eur Spine J,* 2006, 15(3):333–337

Osti OL, Vernon-Roberts B, Moore R et al. 'Annular tears and disc degeneration in the lumbar spine'. *J Bone Joint Surg (Br)* 1992, 74–B:678–82

Schwarzer AC, April CN, Derby R, et al. 'The prevalence and clinical features of internal disc disruption in patients with chronic low back pain'. *Spine.* 1995, 17:1878–1883

Wagner A, Murtagh R, Arrington J, et al. 'Relationship of Schmorl's nodes to vertebral body endplate fractures and acute endplate disk extrusions'. *Am J Neurodrdiol.* 2000, 21:276–281

Weishaupt D, Zanetti M, Hodler J, et al. 'Painful Lumbar Disk Derangement: Relevance of Endplate Abnormalities at MR Imaging'. *Radiology* 2001, 218:420–427

www.chirogeek.com/000_disc_anatomy.htm

http://emedicine.medscape.com/article/1145703-overview#showall

Dry Needling & Acupuncture
Gunn C, Milbrandt W, Little A, et al. 'Dry needling of muscle motor points for chronic low-back pain: a randomized clinical trial with long-term follow-up'. *Spine.* 1980, 5(3): 279–291

Trigkilidas D. 'Acupuncture therapy for chronic lower back pain: a systematic review'. *Annals of the Royal College of Surgeons of England.* 2010, 92(7): 595

Zhang X. 'Acupuncture: Review and analysis of reports on controlled clinical trials'. WHO 1999
https://en.wikipedia.org/wiki/Dry_needling

Exercise therapy

Alfredson H, Pietilä T, Jonsson P, et al. 'Heavy-load eccentric calf muscle training for the treatment of chronic Achilles tendinosis'. *The American Journal of Sports Medicine.* 1998, 26(3): 360–366

Ewert T, Limm H, Wessels T, Rackwitz B, von Garnier K, Freumuth R, Stucki G. 'The comparative effectiveness of a multimodal program versus exercise alone for the secondary prevention of chronic low back pain and disability'. *PM R.* 2009 Sep, 1(9):798–808

Hayden J, Van Tulder M, & Tomlinson G. 'Systematic review: strategies for using exercise therapy to improve outcomes in chronic low back pain'. *Annals of internal medicine.* 2005, 142(9):776–785

McGill S. 'Ultimate Back and Fitness Performance'. Backfitpro incorporated www.backfitpro.com 2007

Nelson BW, O'Reilly E, Miller M, et al. 'The clinical effects of intensive, specific exercise on chronic low-back pain: a controlled study of 895 consecutive patients with one year follow-up'. *Orthopedics.* 1995, 10(10):971–981

Porter RW, Adams MA, Hutton WC. 'Physical activity and the strength of the lumbar spine'. *Spine.* 1989, 14:201–203

Roos E, Engström M, Lagerquist A, et al. 'Clinical improvement after 6 weeks of eccentric exercise in patients with mid-portion Achilles tendinopathy—a randomized trial with 1-year follow-up'. *Scandinavian journal of medicine & science in sports.* 2004, 14(5):286–295.

Van Tulder M, Malmivaara A, Esmail, R, & Koes B. 'Exercise therapy for low back pain: a systematic review within the framework of the Cochrane Collaboration back review group'. *Spine.* 2000, 25(21):2784–2796

Facet Joint problems

Cohen S, Raja S. 'Pathogenesis, diagnosis, and treatment of lumbar zygapophysial (facet) joint pain'. *Anesthesiology.* 2007, 106:591–614

Datta S, Lee M, Falco J, Bryce D, & Hayek S. 'Systematic Assessment of Diagnostic Accuracy and Therapeutic Utility of Lumbar Facet Joint Interventions'. *Pain Physician.* 2009, 12:437–460

Eubanks JD, Lee MJ, Cassinelli E, Ahn NU. 'Prevalence of lumbar facet arthrosis and its relationship to age, sex, and race: An anatomic study of cadaveric specimens'. *Spine.* 2007, 32:2058–2062

Ghormley RK, 'Low back pain with special reference to the articular facets, with presentation of an operative procedure'. *JAMA* 1933, 101:1773–7

References

Kalichman L, Li L, Kim DH, et al. 'Facet joint osteoarthritis and low back pain in the community-based population'. *Spine* 2008, 33:2560–2565

Manchikanti L, Pampati V, Fellows B et al. 'Prevalence of lumbar facet joint pain in chronic low back pain'. *Pain Physician*. 1999, 2:59–64

Mooney V, Roberson J. 'The facet syndrome'. *Clin Orthop* 1976; 115:149–156

Schwarzer A, Aprill C, Derby R, et al. 'Clinical features of patients with pain stemming from the lumbar zygapophysial joints: Is the lumbar facet syndrome a clinical entity?'. *Spine*. 1994;, 9(10):1132–1137

Schwarzer AC, Wang S, Bogduk N et al. 'Prevalence and clinical features of lumbar zygapophysial joint pain: a study in an Australia population with chronic low back pain'. *Ann Rheum Dis*. 1995, 54:100–106

Injections

Alderman D. 'Prolotherapy For Low Back Pain: A reasonable and conservative approach to musculoskeletal low back pain, disc disease, and sciatica'. *Practical Pain Management*. 2007, May

Andreula C, Simonetti L, De Santis F, et al. 'Minimally invasive oxygen-ozone therapy for lumbar disk herniation'. *Am J Neuroradiology*. 2003, 24(5):996–1000

Australian and New Zealand College of Anaesthetists. Faculty of pain management. 'Guidelines for lumbar epidural administration of corticosteroids'. 2010

Carette S, Marcoux S, Truchon R, et al. A 'Controlled Trial of Corticosteroid Injections into Facet Joints for Chronic Low Back Pain'. *N Engl J Med*. 1991, 325:1002–1007

Cholewicke J, McGill S. 'Mechanical stability of the in vivo lumbar spine: implications for injury and chronic low back pain'. *Clinical Biomechanics*. 1996, 11(1):1–15

Couto J, de Castilho E, Menezes P. 'Chemonucleolysis in lumbar disc herniation: A meta-analysis'. *Clinics*. 2007, 62(2):175–80

Dagenais S, Yelland M, Del Mar C, et al. 'Prolotherapy injections for chronic low-back pain'. *Cochrane Database of SystRev*. 2007 (2)

Goupille P, Fitoussi V, Cotty P, et al. 'Injection into the lumbar vertebrae in chronic low back pain. Results in 206 patients'. *Rev Rheum Ed Fr*. 1993, 60(11):797–801.

Guha AR, Debnath UK, D'Souza S. 'Chemonucleolysis revisited: a prospective outcome study in symptomatic lumbar disc prolapse'. *J Spinal Disord Tech*. 2006, 19:167–70

Hildebrandt, J. 'Relevance of nerve blocks in treating and diagnosing low back pain—is the quality decisive?'. *Schmerz (Berlin, Germany)*, 2001, 15(6), 474

Koes B, Scholten R, Mens J, et al. 'Efficacy of epidural steroid injections for low-back pain and sciatica: a systematic review of randomized clinical trials'. *Pain*. 1995, 63:279–288

Kraemer J, Ludwig J, Bickert U, et al. 'Lumbar epidural perineural injection: a new technique'. *Eur Spine J.* 1997, 6:357–361

Lutz G, Vad V, and Wisneski R. 'Fluoroscopic transforaminal lumbar epidural steroids: an outcome study'. *Archives of physical medicine and rehabilitation.* 1998, 79(11):1362–1366

Mayer HM, Wehr M, Brock M, et al. 'Skin testing for chymopapain allergy in chemonucleolysis'. *Surgical Neurology.* 1986, 25(3):283–289

Miller M, Mathews R, Reeves K. 'Treatment of painful advanced internal lumbar disc derangement with intradiscal injection of hypertonic dextrose'. *Pain Physician.* 2006, 9:115–121

Muto M, Andreula C, Leonardi M. 'Treatment of herniated lumbar disc by intradiscal and intraforaminal oxygen-ozone (O2-O3) injection'. *Journal of Neuroradiology.* 2004, 31(3):183–189

Pellicanò G, Martinelli F, Tavanti V, et al. 'The Italian oxygen-ozone therapy federation (FIO) study on oxygen ozone treatment of herniated disc'. *Int J Ozone Ther.* 2007, 6:7–15

Pope M, Frymoyer J, Krag M. 'Diagnosing instability'. *Clinical Orthopaedics and Related Research.* 1992, 296: 60–67.

Steppan J, Meaders T, Muto M, et al. 'A meta-analysis of the effectiveness and safety of ozone treatments for herniated lumbar disc'. *J Vasc Interv Radiol.* 2010, 21:534–548

Sussman BJ. 'Injections of collagenase in the treatment of herniated lumbar disc'. *JAMA.* 1981, 245:730

Yelland M, Glasziou P, Bogduk N, et al. 'Prolotherapy injections, saline injections, and exercises for chronic low-back pain: A randomized trial'. *Spine.* 2003, 29(1):9–16

www.virtualmedicalcentre.com/treatment/nerve-blocks-regional-anaesthesia/49#C4

www.spine-health.com/treatment/injections/injections-back-pain-management

www.spine-health.com/treatment/injections/lumbar-epidural-steroid-injections-low-back-pain-and-sciatica

Instability

O'Sullivan PB. 'Lumbar segmental "instability": clinical presentation and specific stabilizing exercise management'. *Manual Therapy.* 2000, 5(1):2–12

Panjabi M. 'The stabilizing system of the spine. Part 1 and Part 2'. *Journal of Spinal Disorders.* 1992, 5(4): 383–397

Pearcy M, Shepherd J. 'Is there instability in spondylolisthesis?'. *Spine.* 1985, 10:175–177

References

Miscellaneous

Albright J, Allman R, Bonfiglio R, et al. 'Philadelphia Panel Evidence-Based Clinical Practice: Guidelines on Selected Rehabilitation Interventions for low back pain'. *Phys Ther.* 2001, 81:1641–1674

Benz T, Angst F, Aeschlimann A. 'Treatment of chronic pain in Switzerland: scientific evidence'. *Praxis.* 2011 May, 100(10):591–8. PubMed PMID: MEDLINE:21563096.

Bergstrom C, Jensen I, Hagberg J, Busch H, Bergstrom G. 'Effectiveness of different interventions using a psychosocial subgroup assignment in chronic neck and back pain patients: a 10-year follow-up'. *Disability and rehabilitation.* 2012, Epub 2011 Oct, 34(2):110–8

Bogduk N. 'Lumbar dorsal ramus syndrome'. *Med J Aust.* 1980, 2:537–541.

Bolland M, Avenell A, Baron J, et al. 'Effect of calcium supplements on risk of myocardial infarction and cardiovascular events: meta-analysis'. *BMJ.* 2010, 341:c3691

Coulter ID, Hurwitz EL, Adams AH, Genovese BJ, Hays R, Shekelle PG. 'Patients using chiropractors in North America: who are they, and why are they in chiropractic care?'. *Spine.* 2002 Feb, 27(3):291–6; discussion 7–8. PubMed PMID: MEDLINE:11805694.

Cumming R, Cumming S, Nevitt M, et al. 'Calcium intake and fracture risk: Results from the study of osteoporotic fractures'. *Journal of Epidemiology.* 1997, 145(10):926–934

Frisch SA, Widder B. 'Radicular Low Back Pain: Evaluation of Conservative Multimodal Treatment'. *Psychiatr Prax.* 2003 May, 30(Suppl 2):161–166

Furlan A, Imamura M, Dryden T, et al. 'Massage for low-back pain'. *Cochrane Database Syst Rev.* 4.4 (2008)

George JW, Skaggs CD, Thompson PA, Nelson DM, Gavard JA, Gross GA. 'A randomized controlled trial comparing a multimodal intervention and standard obstetrics care for low back and pelvic pain in pregnancy'. *Am J Obstet Gynecol.* 2013 Apr, 208(4):295.e1–7

Hagen KB, Hilde G, Jamtvedt G, Winnem MF. 'The Cochrane review of bed rest for acute low back pain and sciatica'. *Spine.* 2000, 25:2932–2939

Herbert RD, de Noronha M. (2007) 'Stretching to prevent or reduce muscle soreness after exercise'. *Cochrane Database of Systematic Reviews,* Issue 4. Art. No.: CD004577. DOI: 10.1002/14651858.CD004577.pub2

Howitt S, Wong J, & Zabukovec S. 'The conservative treatment of trigger thumb using graston techniques and active release Techniques®'. *The Journal of the Canadian Chiropractic Association.* 2006, 50(4) 249–54

Huynh W, Kiernan M. 'Nerve conduction studies'. *Australian Family Physician.* 2011, 40(9) von Duvillard SP, Braun WA, Markofski M, Beneke R, Leithauser R. 'Fluids and Hydration in Prolonged Endurance Performance'. *Nutrition*. 2004, 20:651–656

Kanis JA and Passmore R. 'Calcium supplementation of the diet–II'. *BMJ*. 1989, 298:205–8

Long D, BenDebba M, Torgenson W. 'Persistent back pain and sciatica in the United States: patient characteristics'. *Journal of Spinal Disorders*. 1996, 9(1): 40–58

Koes BW, Sanders RJ, Tuut MK, Kwaliteitsinstituut voor de Gezondheidszorg CBO. 'The Dutch Institute for Health Care Improvement (CBO) guideline for the diagnosis and treatment of aspecific acute and chronic low back complaints'. *Nederlands tijdschrift voor geneeskunde*. 2004 Feb, 148(7):310–4. PubMed PMID: MEDLINE:15015247.

Kornick C, Kramarich SS, Lamer TJ, et al. 'Complications of lumbar facet radiofrequency denervation'. *Spine*. 2004, 29:1352–1354

Kuhar S, Subhash K, & Chitra J. 'Effectiveness of myofascial release in treatment of plantar fasciitis: An rct'. *Indian Journal of Physiotherapy and Occupational Therapy*. 2007, 1(3):3–9.

Leeuw M, Goossens M, Linton S, et al. 'The fear-avoidance model of musculoskeletal pain: current state of scientific evidence'. *Journal of behavioral medicine*. 2007, 30(1):77–94

Maigne JY, Doursounian L, Chatellier G. 'Causes and Mechanisms of Common Coccydynia: role of BMI and Coccygeal Trauma'. *Spine*. 2000, 25(23):3072–3079

Michealsson A, Melhus H, Warensjo E, et al. 'Long term calcium intake and rates of all cause and cardiovascular mortality: community based prospective longitudinal cohort study'. *BMJ*. 2013, 346:f228.

Micheli LJ, Hall JE, Miller ME. 'Use of modified Boston brace for back injuries in athletes'. *Am J Sports Med*. 1980, 8:5

Nachemson, AL. 'Newest knowledge of low back pain: A critical look'. *Clinical and Orthopedic Related Research,* 1992, 279:8–20.

Niemisto L, Kalso EA, Malmivaara A, et al. 'Radiofrequency denervation for neck and back pain (Review)'. *The Cochran Library*. 2010, 3

Paoloni M, Bernetti A, Fratocchi G, et al. 'Kinesio Taping applied to lumbar muscles influences clinical and electromyographic characteristics in chronic low back pain patients'. *Eur J Phys Rehabil Med*. 2011, 47(2): 237–244

Perez-Lopez F, Brincat M, Tamer Erel C, et al. 'EMAS position statement: Vitamin D and postmenopausal health'. *Maturitas*. 2012, 71(1): 83–88

Porter R. 'Spinal stenosis and neurogenic claudication'. *Spine* 1996, 21(17): 2046–2052

References

Roelofs PD, Deyo RA, Koes BW, Scholten RJ, van Tulder MW. 'Non-steroidal anti-inflammatory drugs for low back pain'. *Cochrane Database Syst Rev.* 2008 Jan 23, (1):CD000396

Hammer, WI. 'The effect of mechanical load on degenerated soft tissue'. *Journal of Bodywork and Movement Therapies.* 2008, 12(3), 246–256

Roland MO. 'A critical review of the evidence for a pain-spasm-pain cycle in spinal disorders'. *Clin Biomech.* 1986, 1:102–109

Rubinstein S, van Middelkoop M, Kuijpers T, et al. 'A systematic review on the effectiveness of complementary and alternative medicine for chronic non-specific low-back pain'. *European Spine Journal.* 2010, 19(8):1213–1228

Rucker D, Allan J, Fick G, et al. 'Vitamin D insufficiency in a population of healthy western Canadians'. *CMAJ.* 2002, 166(12):1517–1524

Russell R. 'The rationale for primary spine care employing biopsychosocial, stratified and diagnosis-based care-pathways at a chiropractic college public clinic: a literature review'. *Chiropractic & Manual Therapies.* 2013, 21:19

Sackett DL, Rosenberg W, Gray JA, et al. 'Evidence based medicine: what it is and what it isn't'. *BMJ* 1996, 312(7023):71–72

Schoeck AP, Mellion ML, Gilchrist JM, et al. 'Safety of nerve conduction studies in patients with implanted cardiac devices'. *Muscle Nerve.* 2007, 35(4):521–4

Shealy CN. 'Facet denervation in the management of back and sciatic pain'. *Clin Orthop Relat Res.* 1976, 115:157–64

van Kleef M, Barendse GA, Kessels A, et al. 'Randomized trial of the radio-frequeny lumbar facet denervation for chronic low back pain'. *Spine.* 1999, 24(18):1937–1942

Vlaeyen J, and Linton S. 'Fear-avoidance and its consequences in chronic musculoskeletal pain: a state of the art'. *Pain.* 2000, 85:317–332

Wainapel S, Thomas A, Kahan B. 'Use of alternative therapies by rehabilitaion outpatients'. *Arch Phys Med Rehab.* 1998, 79:1003–1005

Wang T, Pencina M, Booth S, Jacques P, Ingelsson E, Lanier K, Benjamin E, D'Agostino B, Wolf M & Vasan R. 'Vitamin D Deficiency and Risk of Cardiovascular Disease'. *Journal of the American Heart Association.* 2008, 117:503–511.

Warensjo E, Byberg L, Melhus H, et al. 'Dietary calcium intake and risk of fracture and osteoporosis: prospective longitudinal cohort study'. *BMJ.* 2011, 342:d1473

Williams S, Whatman C, Hume P, et al. 'Kinesio taping in treatment and prevention of sports injuries'. *Sports medicine.* 2012, 42(2):153–164.

Wolsko PM, Eisenberg DM, Davis RB, Kessler R, Phillips RS. 'Patterns and perceptions of care for treatment of back and neck pain: results of a national survey'. *Spine.* 2003 Feb, 28(3):292–7; discussion 8. PubMed PMID: MEDLINE:12567035.

Yamaguchi T, Ishii K. 'Effects of static stretching for 30 seconds and dynamic stretching on leg extension power'. *The Journal of Strength and Conditioning Research*. 2005, 19(3):677–683

www.bigspine.net/injectionsmenu/radio-frequency-denervation.html

www.spine-health.com/conditions/lower-back-pain/coccydynia-tailbone-pain

www.webmd.com/osteoporosis/guide/spinal-compression-fractures-causes

www.medscape.com/viewarticle/442454_2

www.arpansa.gov.au/RadiationProtection/Factsheets/is_CTScansReferrers.cfm

www.hypermobility.org/painandhms.php

Kruszelnicki K.S. 'Knuckle Cracking' www.abc.net.au/science/k2/homework/s95607.htm

www.cigna.com/individualandfamilies/health-and-well-being/hw/medical-tests/electromyogram-and-nerve-conduction-studies-hw213852.html

www.oadortho.com/centers/documents/Dr.MathewSACROILIACJOINT DYSFUNCTION.pdf

The National Sleep Research Project www.abc.net.au/science/sleep/facts.htm

Muscle and Fascia problems

Benjamin M. 'The fascia of the limbs and back—a review'. *J Anat*. 2009, 214(1):1–18

Järvinen TA, Järvinen TL, Kääriäinen M, et al. 'Muscle injuries: biology and treatment'. *Am. J. Sports Med*. 2005, 33;745

Kellgren JH. 'Obserations on referred pain arising from muscle'. *Clin Sci*. 1938, 3:175–190

Richardson CA, Snijdera CJ, Hides JA, et al. 'The relation between the transversus abdominis muscles, sacroiliac joint mechanics and low back pain'. *Spine*. 2002, 27:399–405

Schleip R. 'Fascial plasticity – a new neurobiological explanation: Part 1'. *Journal of Bodywork and Movement Therapies*. 2003, 7(1):11–19

Schleip R, Klinger W. 'Active fascial contractility: Fascia is able to contract and relax in a smooth muscle-like manner and thereby influence biomechanical behavior'. *5th World Congress of Biomechanics*. 2006

Physical therapies

Allen RJ. 'Physical agents used in the management of chronic pain by physical therapists'. *Phys Med Rehabil Clin N Am*. 2006, 17:315–45

Ernst E. 'Massage therapy for low back pain: a systematic review'. *J Pain Symptom Management*. 1999, 17:65–69

French S, Cameron M, Walker B, et al. 'Superficial heat or cold for low back pain'. *Cochrane Database Syst Rev*. 1 (2006)

References

Frey M, Manchikanti L, Ramsin M, et al. 'Spinal Cord Stimulation for Patients with Failed Back Surgery Syndrome: A Systematic Review'. *Pain Physician* 2009, 12:379–397.

Fuentes J, Olivo S, Magee D, et al. 'Effectiveness of interferential current therapy in the management of musculoskeletal pain: a systematic review and meta-analysis'. *Phys Ther.* 2010, 90(9):1219–1238

Ghoname EA, Craig WF, White PF, et al. 'Percutaneous electrical nerve stimulation for low back pain: A randomized crossover study'. *JAMA.* 1999, 281:818–23.

Glaser J, Baltz M, Nietert P, et al. 'Electrical muscle stimulation as an adjunct to exercise therapy in the treatment of nonacute low back pain: a randomized trial'. *The Journal of Pain.* 2001, 2(5):295–300

Hamza M, El-sayed A, White P, et al. 'Effect of the duration of electrical stimulation on the analgesic response in patients with low back pain'. *Anesthesiology.* 1999, 91(6):1622–27

Li LC, Bombardier C. 'Physical therapy management of low back pain: An exploratory survey of therapist approaches'. *Physical Therapy.* 2001, 81(4):1018–28

Marchand S, Charest J, Li J, et al. 'Is TENS purely a placebo effect? A controlled study on chronic low back pain'. *Pain.* 1993, 54:99–106

MacAuley DC. 'Ice therapy: how good is the evidence?'. *International journal of sports medicine.* 2001, 22(05):379–384

Nadler SF, Weingand K. and Kruse RJ. 'The Physiologic Basis and Clinical Applications of Cryotherapy and Thermotherapy for the Pain Practitioner'. *Pain Physician.* 2004, 7:395–399

Poitras S, Brousseau L. 'Evidence-informed management of chronic low back pain with transcutaneous electrical nerve stimulation, interferential current, electrical muscle stimulation, ultrasound, and thermotherapy'. *The Spine Journal.* 2008, 8:226–233

Robertson V, Baker K. 'A review of therapeutic ultrasound: effectiveness studies'. *Physical Therapy.* 2001, 81(7):1339–1350

Sun R, Kim DW, White PF, et al. 'A randomized comparison of non-pharmacologic therapies for the relief of chronic back pain (abstract)'. *Anesth Analg* 1997, 84:S339

Yokoyama M, Sun X, Oku S, et al. 'Comparison of percutaneous electrical nerve stimulation with transcutaneous electrical nerve stimulation for long-term pain relief in patients with chronic low back pain'. *Anesthesia & Analgesia.* 2004, 98(6):1552–1556

Vitiello L, Bonello R, Pollard H. 'The effectiveness of ENAR for the treatment of chronic neck pain in Australian adults: A preliminary single-blinded RCT' *Chiropractic & Osteopathy.* 2007, 15:9 (9 July 2007) http://www.chiroandosteo.com/content/15/1/9

Radiofrequency denervation

Catherine N, Petchprapa CN, Rosenberg ZS, Sconfienza LM, et al. 'MR Imaging of Entrapment Neuropathies of the Lower Extremity : Part 1. The Pelvis and Hip'. *RadioGraphics*. 2010, 30:983–1000

Dvorak J, Panjabi M, Novotny J, et al. 'Clinical validation of functional flexion-extension roentgenograms of the lumbar spine'. *Spine*. 1991, 16(8): 943–950

Hendrich E, Georgen S, Revell A, et al. 'Bone Mineral Density Scan (Bone Densitometry or DEXA Scan)'. *Inside Radiology*. 2009.

Jarvik JG, Hollingworth W, Martin B, et al. 'Rapid magnetic resonance imaging vs radiographs for patients with low back pain; a randomized controlled trial'. *JAMA*. 2003, 289:2810–8

Jensen MC, Brant-Zawadzi MN, Obuchowski N, Modic MT, Malkasian D, Ross JS. 'Magnetic Resonance Imaging of the Lumbar Spine in People without Back Pain'. *The New England Journal of Medicine*. 1994, 2 (331): 69–73

Lurie JD, Birkmeyer NJ, Weinstein JN. 'Rates of advanced spinal imaging and spine surgery'. *Spine*. 2003, 28:616 –20

Rao JK, Kroenke K, Mihaliak KA, et al. 'Can guidelines impact the ordering of magnetic resonance imaging studies by primary care providers for low back pain?'. *Am J Manag Care*. 2002, 8:27–35.

Rubinstein SM, van Tulder M. 'A best-evidence review of diagnostic procedures for neck and low-back pain'. *Best Pract Res Clin Rheumatol*. 2008, 22:471–482

Sanders R. 'Radiation expert warns of danger from overuse of medical X-rays, claiming they're responsible for many cancer and heart disease deaths'. *Public Affairs*. 1999, (510) 642–3734

Walker III J, El Abd O, Isaac Z, et al. 'Discography in practice: a clinical and historical review'. *Curr Rev Musculoskelet Med*. 2008, 1:69–83

Walsh TR, Weinstein JN, Spratt KF, et al. 'Lumbar discography in normal subjects. A controlled, prospective study'. *J Bone Joint Surg Am*. 1990, 72:1081–1088

Spinal manipulation

Assendelft W, Morton S, Yu E, et al. 'Spinal manipulative therapy for low-back pain'. *Cochrane database syst Rev 1*. 2004(1)

Cassidy J, Kirkaldy-Willis WH, McGregor M. 'Spinal manipulation for the treatment of chronic low back and leg pain: an observational trial'. In: Buerger AA, Greenman PE, eds. *Empirical Approaches to the Validation of Manipulative Therapy*. Springfiled, IL: Charles C Thomas; 1985.

Cassidy JD, Porter GE, Kirkaldy-Willis WH. 'Manipulative management of back pain patients with spondylolisthesis'. *J Can Chiro Assoc*. 1978, 22:15

References

Bronfort G, Evans R, Anderson AV, Svendsen KH, Bracha Y, Grimm RH. 'Spinal manipulation, medication, or home exercise with advice for acute and subacute neck pain: a randomized trial'. *Annals of internal medicine.* 2012 Jan, 156(1 Pt 1):1–10

Haldeman S, Rubinstein SM. 'Cauda equina syndrome in patients undergoing manipulation of the lumbar spine'. *Spine* 1992, 17(12):1469

Hurley D, McDonough S, Dempster M, et al. 'A randomized clinical trial of manipulative therapy and interferential therapy for acute low back pain'. *Spine.* 2004, 29(20):2207–2216

Rajadurai V, Murugan K. 'Spinal manipulative therapy for low back pain: A systematic review'. *Physical Therapy Reviews.* 2009, 14(4):260–271

Rubinstein S, van Middelkoop M, Assendelft W, et al. 'Spinal Manipulative Therapy for Chronic Low-Back Pain'. *Spine.* 2011, 36(13):E825–E846

Snelling N. 'Spinal manipulation in patients with disc herniation: A critical review of risk and benefit'. *Intern J of Ortho Med.* 2006, 9(3):77–84

Surgery

Andersson G, Mekhail N, Block J. 'Treatment of intractable discogenic low back pain: A systematic review of spinal fusion and intradiscal electrothermal therapy (IDET)'. *Paiin Physician.* 2006, 9:237–248.

Andreula C, Muto M, Leonardi M. 'Interventional spinal procedures'. *Eur J Radiol.* 2004, 50:112–119

Bouillet R. 'Treatment of sciatica, a comparative survey of complications of surgical treatment and nucleolysis with chymopapain'. *Clin Orthop Relat Res.* 1990, 251:144–52

Deyo A, Nachemson A, Mirza S. 'Spinal-fusion surgery—the case for restraint'. *N Engl J Med.* 2004, 350(7):722–726

German JW, Adamo MA, Hoppenot RG, et al. 'Perioperative results following lumbar discectomy: comparison of minimally invasive discectomy and standard microdiscectomy'. *Neurosurg Focus.* 2008, 25:E20

Helthoff KB, Burton CV. 'CT evaluation of the failed back surgery syndrome'. *Orthop Clin North Am* 1985, 16:417–44

Johnsson KE, Uden A, Rosen I. 'The effect of compression on the natural course of spinal stenosis: a comparison of surgically treated and untreated patients'. *Spine.* 1991, 16:615–619.

Kostelianetz M, Espersen JO, Halaburt H, Miletic T. 'Predictive value of clinical and surgical findings in patients with lumbago-sciatica. A prospective study (Part I)'. *Acta Neurochir.* 1984, 73:67–76

Lau D, Han SJ, Lee J, et al. 'Minimally invasive compared to open microdiscectomy for lumbar disc herniation'. *J Clin Neurosci.* 2010, doi:10.1016/j.jocn.2010.04.040

Markwalder TM, Battaglia M. 'Failed back surgery of complications of surgical treatment and nucleolysis with chymopapain'. *Clin Orthop Relat Res.* 1990, 251:144–52

Österman H, Seitsalo S, Karppinen J, et al. 'Effectiveness of Microdiscectomy for Lumbar Disc Herniation: A Randomized Controlled Trial With 2 Years of Follow-up'. *Spine.* 2006, 31(21):2409–2414

Pauza KJ, Howell S, Dreyfuss P, et al. 'A randomized, placebo-controlled trial of intradiscal electrothermal therapy for the treatment of discogenic low back pain'. *Spine.* 2004, 4:27–35

Porchet F, Bartanusz V, Kleinstueck FS, et al. 'Microdiscectomy compared with standard discectomy: an old problem revisited with new outcome measures within the framework of a spine surgical registry'. *Eur Spine J.* 2009, 3:360–6

Porter RW. 'Spinal surgery and alleged medical negligence'. *J R Coll Surg Edinb.* 1997, 42:376–80.

Schaeren S, Broger I, Jeannere B. 'Minimum Four-Year Follow-up of Spinal Stenosis With Degenerative Spondylolisthesis Treated With Decompression and Dynamic Stabilization'. *Spine.* 2008, 33(18): pp E636 –E642

Skaf G., Bouclaous C, Alaraj A, et al. 'Clinical outcome of surgical tratment of failed back surgery syndrome'. *Surgical Neurology* 2005, 64(6):483–488

Talbot, L. 'Failed back surgery syndrome'. *BMJ* 2003, 327:985–987

Turner Ersek M, Herron L, et al. 'Patient outcomes after lumbar spinal fusions'. *JAMA* 1992, 268:907–911

Voormolen, MHJ, et al. 'Percutaneous vertebroplasty compared with optimal pain medication treatment: short-term clinical outcome of patients with subacute or chronic painful osteoporotic vertebral compression fractures. The VERTOS study'. *American journal of neuroradiology.* 2007, 28(3): 555–560

Waguespack, A, Schofferman, J, Slosar, P, et al. 'Etiology of long-term failures of lumbar spine surgery'. *Pain Medicine.* 2002, 3:18–22

www.spine-health.com/treatment/spinal-fusion/lumbar-spinal-fusion-surgery

http://sosspine.com/spinal_fusion_surgery

www.spine-health.com/treatment/back-surgery/idet-a-new-procedure-discogenic-back-pain-management

www.spine-health.com/treatment/back-surgery/microdiscectomy-micro decompression-spine-surgery

www.medscape.com/viewarticle/762967?sssdmh=dm1.780699&src=nldne

Traction

Clarke JA, van Tulder MW, Blomberg SEI, et al. 'Traction for low-back pain with or without sciatica'. *Cochrane database syst Rev.* 2007(2)

Krause M, Refshauge K, Dessen M, et al. 'Lumbar spine traction: evaluation of effects and recommended application for treatment'. *Manual Therapy.* 2000, 5(2):72–81

References

Saunders D. 'Lumbar traction'. *JOSPT.* 1979, 1(1):36–45

Twomey L. 'Sustained lumbar traction: An experimental study of long spine segments'. *Spine.* 1985, 10(2):

van der Heijden G, Beurskens A, Koes B, et al. 'The efficacy of traction for back and neck pain: A systematic, blinded review of randomized clinical trial methods'. *Phys Ther.* 1995, 75:93–104

Trigger point therapy

de las Peñas C, Sohrbeck Campo M, Fernández Carnero J, et al. 'Manual therapies in myofascial trigger point treatment: a systematic review'. *Journal of bodywork and movement therapies.* 2005, 9(1):27–34

Harden RN, Bruehl SP, Gass S, et al. 'Signs and symptoms of the myofascial pain syndrome: a national survey of pain management providers'. *Clin J Pain.* 2000, 16:64–72

McPartland J. 'Travell Trigger Points—Molecular and Osteopathic Perspectives'. *J Am Osteopath Assoc.* 2004, 104(6):244–249

Vernon H, & Schneider M. 'Chiropractic management of myofascial trigger points and myofascial pain syndrome: a systematic review of the literature'. *Journal of manipulative and physiological therapeutics.* 2009, 32(1):14–24

Books

Belanger AY. *Evidence based guide to therapeutic physical agents.* Philadelphia: Lippincott Williams & Wilkins; 2002

Bogduk N. *Clinical and Radiological Anatomy of the Lumbar Spine.* 5th ed. 2012 Edinburgh: Churchill Livingstone

Cameron MH. *Physical agents in rehabilitation: from research to practice.* Philadelphia: W.B. Saunders; 2003

Davies C, Simons D, & Davies A. *The trigger point therapy workbook: your self-treatment guide for pain relief.* 2004. New Harbinger Publications Incorporated

Dilorenzo, DJ and Bronzino, JD. *Neuroengineering.* 2008. CRC Press. (Chapter 7)

Fortanasce V, Gutkind D, Watkins R. *End back & neck pain.* 2012. Human Kinetics; 2012

Jamison J. *Clinical guide to Nutrition & Dietary Supplements in Disease Management.* 2003. Churchill Livingstone

Levangie P & Norkin C. *Joint Structure and Function: A Comprehensive Analysis.* 3rd ed. 2001. F.A. Davis Company

Lee, P. 'Modalities'. In *Rehab Clinical Pocket Guide.* 2013 (pp. 305–331). Springer New York

Liebenson C. *Rehabilitation of the Spine*. 2nd ed. 2007. Sydney: Lippincott Williams and Wilkins

Maxey L, and Magnusson J. *Rehabilitation for the Postsurgical Orthopedic Patient*. 2001. Mosby, St. Louis.

McFarland C. and Burkhart D. *Rehabilitation Protocols for Surgical and Nonsurgical Procedures: Lumbar Spine*: 2001. North Atlantic Books, Berkeley, CA

McGill S. *Ultimate Back and Fitness Performance*. 2007. Elsevier

Middleditch, A & Oliver J. *Functional Anatomy of the Spine*. 2nd ed. 2004. Elsevier

Myers, T. *Anatomy Trains: myofascial meridians for manual and movement therapists*. 2nd Ed. 2009. Churchill Livingstone Elsevier

Rachman, S. *Anxiety*. 1998. Psychological Press, Hove

Schleip R, Findley T, Chaitow L, et al. *Fascia: The tensional network of the human body*. 2012. Churchill Livingstone

Souza TA. *Differential Diagnosis and Management for the Chiropractor: Protocols and Algorithms*. 3rd ed. 2005. Jones and Bartlett Publishers, Sudbury, MA

Strax TE, Gonzalez P, Cuccurullo S. 'Physical Modalities'. In: Cuccurullo S, editor. *Physical Medicine and Rehabilitation Board Review*. 2004. New York: Demos Medical Publishing

Travell JG, Simons DG. *Myofascial Pain and Dysfunction: The Trigger Point Manual: The Upper Extremities*. Vol.1. 1983. Baltimore, Md: Williams & Wilkins

Travell JG, Simons DG. *Myofascial Pain and Dysfunction: The Trigger Point Manual: The Lower Extremities*. Vol. 2. 1983. Baltimore, Md: Williams & Wilkins

Yochum, TR, Rowe L. *Essentials of Skeletal Radiology*. Vol 1. Third Edition. 2005. Lippincott Williams and Wilkins

Wyss J, Patel A. *Therapeutic Programs for Musculoskeletal Disorders*. 2012. pp. 355–360 Demosmedical

Acknowledgements

The authors sincerely appreciate the following professionals and friends who helped make this book possible by contributing to the many tasks involved: Professor Peter Tuchin wrote the chapter on back pain and the workplace, Mr David de la Harpe contributed to the section on surgical treatments, Dr Curtis Rigney reviewed the exercise colour section, Dr Hazel Jenkins provided expertise on medical imaging, Dr Martin Harvey contributed the foreword to this book and Martha Bonello was a model for some of the photos in the colour section.

We also greatly value the athletes' contribution to this book by providing their personal experiences in dealing with back pain—Drew Ginn, Anna Meares, Dan O'Brien and Rener Gracie.

We would also like to thank the team at Allen & Unwin who were enthusiastic about this project right from the very start, especially Lizzy Walton, Melissa Faulkner and Kathryn Knight, who were an absolute delight to work with.

About the authors

Adam Gavine has a Bachelor of Human Kinetics (Hons), Windsor University, Ontario, and a Master of Chiropractic, Macquarie University, Sydney. An active Sydney-based clinician, Adam has sought further qualifications in chiropractic care for pregnancy, spinal rehabilitation, foot biomechanics, running biomechanics and dry needling.

Adam is also one of only a handful of fully qualified Active Release Techniques (ART) providers in Australia to be certified in Upper, Lower and Spine protocols. ART is a very effective myofascial release technique that works on soft tissues of the body to restore strength, flexibility and function.

Growing up Adam played many sports: ice hockey, volleyball, tennis, and soccer. However, he eventually decided to focus on one sport in which he excelled: athletics. Adam competed as a multi-event track and field athlete for ten years. During this time Adam represented Canada as a junior in the decathlon, was provincial interuniversity champion in the pentathlon, and placed fifth at the Canadian Interuniversity Sports Championships while competing for the University of Windsor. Adam's diverse sporting background, and his experience working with semi-professional football and basketball teams as well as treating several members of the Canadian Olympic team, has provided him with a unique understanding of the level of commitment and the demands athletes place on their bodies.

Adam was recently elected as an executive board member of the Chiropractic and Osteopathic College of Australasia (COCA), which is the second largest chiropractic association in Australia.

Rod Bonello is an internationally respected academic, scientist and author. He achieved a world first in chiropractic education by creating the first university-based chiropractic program in 1990. Since that time seven other universities have followed his lead, most of them adopting the new educational model created by Professor Bonello. In addition, a number of physiotherapy and podiatry programs have also used the same model. He became Head of Department at Macquarie University in Sydney, a position he held for over ten years. Currently he is an Honorary Associate of Murdoch University.

While Professor Bonello has educated over half the chiropractors in Australia he has also provided lectures to multidisciplinary groups including medical professionals and physiotherapists locally and internationally.

He has been in high demand as an expert in his field in medico-legal cases and peer professional review. He has also appeared on national and state media to explain new advances in spinal pain management. He has appeared on *A Current Affair*, five sequential sessions of Channel Ten News in Sydney, and twice on ABC Radio.

Professor Bonello has presented his research at conferences on four continents and has been the principal supervisor for ten PhD research projects and contributed to many others. He has organised and moderated scientific conferences in this field and has authored over sixty peer-reviewed, scientific publications on back pain, sports injury, various health disorders (such as Attention Deficit Disorder, jaw problems, thyroid problems, and shoulder problems) and on the health care industry. He is a member of the editorial board of three international journals.

He was a member of the Board of the Australian Spinal Research Foundation for fourteen years, serving as Honorary Secretary for ten. He has been awarded two Fellowships and has been an Australian Chiropractor of the Year.